State Laws Relating to Breast Cancer

Division of Cancer Prevention and Control

Legislative Summary
January 1949 to May 2000

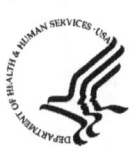

U.S. DEPARTMENT OF HEALTH AND HUMAN SERVICES
Centers for Disease Control and Prevention

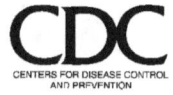

CONTENTS

This document was prepared July 2000 by:

Office of Program and Policy Information
Division of Cancer Prevention and Control
National Center for Chronic Disease Prevention
and Health Promotion
Centers for Disease Control and Prevention
4770 Buford Highway, NE (Mailstop K-64)
Atlanta, Georgia 30341

EXECUTIVE SUMMARY

The following is a digest of significant statutes affecting breast cancer from the 50 states and the District of Columbia. These statutes reflect the past and present concerns of legislatures regarding breast cancer. Most statutes addressing breast cancer are of recent (post-1980) origin, but research has identified relevant laws as far back as 1949. For example, a 1949 Alabama law required that the state Board of Health's program for indigent cancer sufferers include examinations for breast cancer (see p.17).

Over the past two decades, state legislatures have addressed a number of different areas relating to breast cancer. In the early 1980s, several states mandated that health insurers reimburse policyholders for breast reconstruction or prosthetics incident to mastectomy. A decade later, with the increasing incidence of breast cancer, the legislative focus turned to prevention. All but one state (Utah) now requires that health insurance policies offer reimbursement for mammography screening.

This summary covers all legislation enacted between January 1949 and May 2000. The statutes were identified and obtained by searching LEXIS-NEXIS, an online commercial information service. Statutes relevant to the following categories are included in this report:

- Breast Cancer Screening and Education Programs
- Reimbursement for Breast Cancer Screening
- Reimbursement for Breast Reconstruction or Prosthesis
- Accreditation of Facilities and Technologies
- Alternative Therapies
- Reimbursement for Chemotherapy and/or Bone Marrow Transplants
- Income Tax Checkoff for Breast Cancer Funds
- Reimbursement for Length of Stay/Inpatient Care Following Mastectomy

ANALYSIS OF RESULTS BY MAJOR BREAST CANCER STATUTE CATEGORY

CDC funds the National Breast and Cervical Early Detection Program in all states, the District of Columbia, 6 U.S. territories, and 12 American Indian/Alaska Native organizations. The participating entities support this detection program with $1 of their own funds for every $3 provided by CDC. Many states in addition have passed various legislation, such as the following, related to cervical cancer.

Breast Cancer Screening and Education Programs
Twenty-four states have created breast cancer screening and education programs by statute. These public health programs address breast cancer control through activities such as mammography for low-income or underserved populations, distribution of brochures or standardized summaries of treatment methods, operation of referral services and cancer registries, and creation of advisory councils.

Reimbursement for Breast Cancer Screening
Most jurisdictions have traditionally required insurance coverage for preventive care in general. In 1981, only one state (Illinois) specifically required that insurers cover mammograms. By the end of May 2000, the District of Columbia and all states except Utah had mandated health insurance reimbursement for breast cancer screening using mammography for all women covered by health insurance. These statutes, most of which were enacted during or after 1989, typically apply to accident and health insurers, health maintenance organizations (HMOs), and hospital and medical service corporations ("the Blues"). Several states have separate provisions for public employee health insurance plans or Medicare supplement insurance. Some states require mammography coverage only if the insurer also covers mastectomies or prosthetic devices. By statute, mandated mammography coverage specifically applies to Medicaid or comparable medical assistance programs in eight jurisdictions (Alabama, California, the District of Columbia, Illinois, Montana, Nebraska, New Mexico, and Ohio). By statute or agency policy, Medicaid or public assistance programs in all 50 states and the District of Columbia cover mammography screening for breast cancer either routinely or upon a physician's recommendation.

The abstracts included in this digest indicate age and frequency requirements for mammograms. A majority of states mandate coverage for a baseline mammogram for women aged 35 to 39, mammograms every 2 years for women in their forties, and annual mammograms for those aged 50 years and older. In addition, many state mandates address "women at risk." These mandates typically require coverage of screening mammography annually or upon a physician's recommendation for any woman who has a personal or family history of breast cancer, or who has not given birth by age 30.

Most states' coverage mandates include quality assurance requirements for mammography. These provisions typically require that the equipment used be specifically designed and dedicated for mammography. Coverage may also include a physician's interpretation of the results.

Reimbursement for Breast Reconstruction or Prosthesis
Twenty-eight states require health insurance reimbursement for post-mastectomy breast reconstruction or prosthesis. Some states require coverage of reconstruction or prosthesis only if the insurer also covers surgical services for mastectomies. In addition to reconstruction of the diseased breast, many states require reimbursement for reconstructive surgery on the nondiseased breast, performed in order to achieve symmetry following a mastectomy.

Accreditation of Facilities and Technologists
Seventeen jurisdictions have enacted laws specifically addressing accreditation of facilities and technologists. The earliest of these provisions went into effect in 1989 in Michigan and Rhode Island. These statutes specifically provide for the licensing or certification of mammography facilities and operating personnel and are in addition to or in lieu of statutes governing radiology generally.

The provisions often explicitly incorporate American College of Radiology Mammography Accreditation Program guidelines or reference the Mammography Quality Standards Act of 1992.

Informed Decision-Making Concerning Alternative Therapies
In statutes dating primarily from the mid-1980s, 14 states require that physicians inform patients of the advantages, disadvantages, and risks of medically viable alternative therapies for the treatment of breast cancer. These laws may require use of a standardized written summary prepared by a state agency or the posting of signs outlining these alternatives. Some states also require the use of written consent for treatment forms signed by all breast cancer patients, verifying that they have received the information mandated by these statutes.

Reimbursement for Chemotherapy and/or Bone Marrow Transplants
Ten states require insurers to offer coverage for chemotherapy and/or bone marrow transplants for the treatment of breast cancer. Eight of these 10 laws have come into effect since 1993. The statutes typically include quality assurance provisions relating to treatment facilities and protocols and require that coverage levels be no less favorable than for other services.

Note: Although they have not been proven effective against breast cancer in the long-term, bone marrow transplants are offered as a treatment option for breast cancer and are the subject of legislation in many states, so legislation on this topic is included in this report.

Income Tax Checkoff for Breast Cancer Funds
Since 1993, nine states have enacted laws that enable taxpayers to contribute to state breast cancer funds via income tax checkoffs. Contributions can be designated on individual or corporate income tax returns. The funds are used to support breast cancer research or screening and education programs within the state.

Reimbursement for Length of Stay/Inpatient Care Following Mastectomy
Seventeen states have enacted laws relating to reimbursement for specified lengths of inpatient stay in the hospital following mastectomy and/or lumpectomy and lymph node dissection. Several of these laws also mandate reimbursement for outpatient visits following hospital discharge if a shorter length of stay is chosen by the patient in consultation with his or her attending physician.

Statutes on Other Breast Cancer Topics
Less common statutory provisions relating to breast cancer address the following:

- Restrictions on the denial of insurance coverage for breast cancer survivors (Connecticut, Florida, New York, and Washington).
- Informed consent for the treatment of breast cancer (Louisiana, Maine, Montana, Pennsylvania, and Virginia).

- Funds for breast cancer research, screening, diagnosis, and treatment (Arkansas, California, Illinois, Kentucky, Nebraska, Rhode Island, and West Virginia). One state (Louisiana) has established a Breast Cancer Control Program with funds derived from the Tobacco Settlement (see p. 89).
- Reporting requirements for mammography services (Maine).
- Breast cancer early detection instruction in public schools (Indiana, Louisiana, Massachusetts, and New York).
- Grant awards for breast cancer early detection and research (New York).
- Special license plates supporting breast cancer screening and research (Alabama, New York, Oklahoma, and Virginia).
- Advertising of mammography services (Oklahoma).
- Breast Cancer Treatment Programs (California).
- Mammography Registry (Vermont).

Tables I through III provide a snapshot breast cancer legislation by enactor (state or District of Columbia). Table I shows breast cancer laws by category and enactor. Table II provides a snapshot of breast cancer laws by enactor, category of breast cancer law, and year the law was enacted. Table III shows laws relating to reimbursement for breast cancer screening by enactor and type of provision enacted.

TABLE I (PART I)
BREAST CANCER LAWS BY CATEGORY AND ENACTOR
(JANUARY 1949 TO MAY 2000)

Enactor	Category of Breast Cancer Law							
	Breast Cancer Screening and Education Programs	Reimbursement for Breast Cancer Screening	Reimbursement for Breast Reconstruction or Prosthesis	Accreditation of Facilities and Technologists	Alternative Therapies	Reimbursement for Chemotherapy and/or Bone Marrow Transplants	Income Tax Checkoff for Breast Cancer Funds	Length of Stay/ Inpatient Care Following Mastectomy
Alabama	M	M	M					
Alaska		M						
Arizona		M	M	M				
Arkansas	M	M	M	M				M
California	M	M	M	M	M		M	M
Colorado	M	M		M				
Connecticut	M	M	M				M	
Delaware		M					M	
District of Columbia		M						
Florida	M	M	M	M	M			M
Georgia	M	M				M		M
Hawaii		M						
Idaho		M		M				
Illinois	M	M	M	M			M	M
Indiana		M	M					
Iowa		M		M				
Kansas	M	M			M			
Kentucky	M	M	M		M	M		
Louisiana	M	M	M		M		M	
Maine		M	M		M			M
Maryland	M	M	M	M	M			
Massachusetts	M	M		M		M		
Michigan	M	M	M	M	M			
Minnesota		M			M	M		
Mississippi		M						
Missouri		M	M	M		M		

Enactor	Category of Breast Cancer Law							
	Breast Cancer Screening and Education Programs	Reimbursement for Breast Cancer Screening	Reimbursement for Breast Reconstruction or Prosthesis	Accreditation of Facilities and Technologists	Alternative Therapies	Reimbursement for Chemotherapy and/or Bone Marrow Transplants	Income Tax Checkoff for Breast Cancer Funds	Reimbursement for Length of Stay/ Inpatient Care Following Mastectomy
Montana		M	M		M	M		M
Nebraska	M	M						
Nevada		M	M	M				
New Hampshire		M				M		
New Jersey	M	M	M			M	M	M
New Mexico		M						M
New York	M	M	M		M		M	M
North Carolina		M	M					M
North Dakota		M						
Ohio	M	M						
Oklahoma	M	M	M				M	M
Oregon		M						
Pennsylvania		M	M	M	M		M	M
Rhode Island		M	M	M				M
South Carolina		M	M					M
South Dakota	M	M						
Tennessee		M	M			M		
Texas	M	M	M	M	M			M
Utah	M			M				
Vermont		M						
Virginia		M	M		M	M		M
Washington		M	M					
West Virginia	M	M						
Wisconsin	M	M	M					
Wyoming		M						

TABLE II (PART I)
MAJOR BREAST CANCER STATUTES BY STATE, CATEGORY OF STATUTE, AND YEAR ENACTED (1980 TO 2000)

Category of Statute	1980*	1981	1982	1983	1984	1985	1986	1987	1988	1989	1990	1991	1992	1993	1994	1995	1996	1997	1998	1999	2000	Total
Breast Cancer Screening and Education Programs	AL CA GA NY	CA NJ			KY		MD MI		CO	IL MI NY	KY	IL SD TX WI	UT WV	KS NJ	CA OK	FL MD NY	CT MD	AR MA	MD NE OH	GA	LA NE	24
Reimbursement for Breast Cancer Screening		IL	NC					HI MA TX	AZ CA CT KS MN RI	IN MI NV NH ND OK TN WV	AR KY MO NM NY SD VA WA WI	AK DC IL IA ME MD MT NJ VT	CO GA ID IN LA NC OH PA	OR		FL NE	WV	AL ME NM	DE MD SC WY	IN MS		50
Reimbursement for Breast Reconstruction or Prosthesis	CA	AZ IL		MI NV NJ WA	NY VA			FL			WI	CT				ME	MD	AR CT IN OK RI TN TX	KY LA MO MT NC PA VA	MD SC	AL	28

* This category includes statutes in effect by 1980.

TABLE II (PART II)

MAJOR BREAST CANCER STATUTES BY STATE, CATEGORY OF STATUTE, AND YEAR ENACTED
1980-2000

State and Year Enacted

Category of Statute	1980	1981	1982	1983	1984	1985	1986	1987	1988	1989	1990	1991	1992	1993	1994	1995	1996	1997	1998	1999	2000	Total
Accreditation of Facilities and Technologists									MI RI			FL IL NV	IA MD MA MO PA UT	CA CO ID	AZ TX	AR UT						17
Alternative Therapies	CA		MN		FL KY PA VA		MD MI		ME			TX		KS					MT NY		LA	13
Reimbursement for Chemotherapy and/or Bone Marrow Transplants				NJ	VA									NH	MA	GA MN VA	KY MO TN	VA	MT			10
Income Tax Checkoff for Breast Cancer Funds														IL	CA OK	NJ	DE NY	CT PA		LA		9
Reimbursement for Length of Stay/Inpatient Care Following Mastectomy					NY VA													AR FL IL NJ NM NC OK RI TX	ME MT PA VA	CA GA SC		17

TABLE III (PART I)
STATE LAWS ON REIMBURSEMENT FOR BREAST CANCER SCREENING
BY ENACTOR AND TYPE OF PROVISION ENACTED
(JANUARY 1949 TO MAY 2000)

Enactor	Type of Provision Provided					
	Mandates Reimbursement for Breast Cancer Screening	Mandate Applies to Medicaid or Public Assistance	Mandate References Public Employee Health Benefits	Mandate Applies to Medicare Supplement Insurance	Age and Frequency Provision	"Woman at Risk" Provision
Alabama	M	M			M	
Alaska	M				M	M
Arizona	M				M	
Arkansas	M				M	M
California	M	M			M	
Colorado	M				M	M
Connecticut	M			M	M	
Delaware	M				M	M
District of Columbia	M	M				
Florida	M				M	M
Georgia	M				M	M
Hawaii	M				M	M
Idaho	M				M	
Illinois	M	M	M		M	
Indiana	M		M	M	M	M
Iowa	M				M	
Kansas	M					
Kentucky	M				M	
Louisiana	M		M		M	
Maine	M				M	
Maryland	M	M		M	M	
Massachusetts	M				M	
Michigan	M				M	
Minnesota	M			M		
Mississippi	M				M	
Missouri	M				M	M
Montana	M	M			M	

TABLE III (PART II)
STATE LAWS ON REIMBURSEMENT FOR BREAST CANCER SCREENING
BY ENACTOR AND TYPE OF PROVISION ENACTED
(JANUARY 1949 TO MAY 2000)

Enactor	Type of Provision Enacted					
	Mandates Reimbursement for Breast Cancer Screening	Mandate Applies to Medicaid or Public Assistance	Mandate References Public Employee Health Benefits	Mandate Applies to Medicare Supplement Insurance	Age and Frequency Provision	"Woman at Risk" Provision
Nebraska	M	M			M	M
Nevada	M				M	
New Hampshire	M				M	
New Jersey	M				M	
New Mexico	M	M			M	
New York	M				M	M
North Carolina	M		M		M	M
North Dakota	M				M	
Ohio	M	M	M		M	M
Oklahoma	M				M	
Oregon	M				M	M
Pennsylvania	M				M	
Rhode Island	M					
South Carolina	M				M	
South Dakota	M				M	
Tennessee	M				M	
Texas	M			M	M	
Utah						
Vermont	M				M	
Virginia	M		M		M	
Washington	M		M			
West Virginia	M		M		M	
Wisconsin	M				M	
Wyoming	M					

CDC's National Breast and Cervical Cancer Early Detection Program: A Federally Mandated Program

CDC is working under federal mandate and with states, tribes, U.S. territories, and other partners to conduct, fund, and support activities and programs for the prevention of cervical cancer. CDC recognizes that legislation is a very important public health tool in the fight against cervical cancer; therefore, as a service to its partners, CDC has compiled this digest of significant statutes regarding cervical cancer. This section contains a description of CDC's federally mandated National Breast and Cervical Cancer Early Detection Program.

In 1990, federal legislation established CDC's National Breast and Cervical Cancer Early Detection Program (NBCCEDP). The program's goal is to increase the early detection of breast and cervical cancer. The program provides breast and cervical cancer screening exams and referral services to underserved women, including those who are older, have low incomes, or are members of racial and ethnic minority groups. Programs also support public education, professional education, quality assurance, surveillance, program evaluation, and administration. The federal law created a comprehensive approach to controlling cervical cancer.

The program operates in all 50 states, the District of Columbia, 6 U.S. territories, and 12 American Indian/Alaska Native organizations. Screening services provided by the program include clinical breast examinations, mammograms, pelvic examinations, and Pap tests. Post-screening diagnostic services, such as surgical consultation and biopsy, are also funded by the program to ensure that all women with abnormal screening results receive timely and adequate diagnostic evaluation and treatment referrals.

A budget of more than $160 million in FY 2000 is enabling CDC to increase education and outreach programs for women and health care providers, improve quality assurance measures for screening, provide enhanced case management services, and improve access to screening and follow-up services.

The NBCCEDP has made significant progress in building state partnerships to serve women. Five states (Connecticut, Nebraska, New York, Rhode Island, and West Virginia) have created federally-funded cervical cancer early detection programs by statute. State health agencies contract with a broad range of provider agencies, based upon available resources, to deliver screening services. In Nebraska, for example, the state contracts directly with health clinics of Nebraska's federally recognized Native American tribes, Indian health organizations, or other public health organizations that have a substantial Native American clientele to provide cervical cancer screening and early detection services targeted to Native American populations (see page 35). The success of NBCCEDP over the past decade has contributed to the growing pressure on state legislatures to focus more attention on cervical cancer prevention and control.

Nationwide Program Accomplishments (1990 through September 1999)
- **Nearly 1.2 million mammograms provided.**
- **More than 1.3 million Pap tests provided.**
- **More than 7,300 breast cancers diagnosed.**
- **More than 37,000 precancerous cervical lesions diagnosed.**
- **More than 600 cervical cancers diagnosed.**

Research

CDC conducts and supports research through this program, providing information that can be used to protect women from breast and cervical cancer in all other arenas. For example, available data suggest mammography rescreening rates are low among women in the program, despite their access to free examinations. Comparing mammograms taken over time for each woman is essential for early detection of changes in the breast, particularly those that might lead to cancer. CDC is conducting a study to determine valid, precise estimates of mammography rescreening rates in the program and the risk factors that contribute to women not being rescreened on schedule. This information can be used to identify the women most at risk of not being rescreened and to help overcome the identified barriers and risk factors.

Programs

CDC works with health care professionals and organizations, human services and voluntary organizations, academia, and health agencies to provide effective outreach programs. CDC funds a strong and effective network of partners who are well-positioned in communities at risk. These partners have developed projects that are focused on underserved populations and cover a wide range of public and professional education interventions. For example, many projects are involved with developing low-literacy, bilingual, and culturally appropriate educational materials that are used in diverse training and outreach programs and educational campaigns. The various interventions used by the different projects contribute to the common goal of increasing access to and use of screening services among priority populations.

Quality Control
- CDC provides national guidance and support to ensure that screening-related professional and medical services incorporate current techniques and best practices.
- CDC provides screening and diagnostic guidelines to all funded programs and assists them in evaluating their clinical services.
- CDC distributes case management procedures and policies to all participating programs.

Training

Through professional education services, the program has helped a wide range of health care professionals—including physicians, nurses, radiology technologists, and cytologists—better understand and perform their key roles in the early detection of breast and cervical cancer.

For example,

- CDC's national training center for cancer detection and prevention has recently developed a self-study packet with a videotape to help providers—particularly those in rural areas—improve follow-up of women who have abnormal screening results from clinical breast examinations and mammograms. The training center also offers Native American nurses "Native Web" training to enhance their clinical breast examination skills.

- Professional education opportunities are also offered through the program's state, tribal, and territorial programs. For example, the Kentucky Cancer Program offers a self-study kit to help primary care physicians increase and improve routine breast and cervical cancer screenings. The program features a videotape discussing communication strategies, physical examination recommendations and techniques, risk management, and office reminder systems.

LIST OF STATUTES BY STATE AND NUMBER

Alabama

Code of Ala. § 22-13-6
Code of Ala. §§ 27-50-1 to 27-50-7
2000 AL SB 559
Code of Ala. § 32-6-591

Alaska

Alaska Stat. § 21.42.375

Arizona

A.R.S. §§ 20-826(I), 20-934(G), 20-1057(J), 20-1342(A)(10), 20-1402(A)(6), 20-1404(H)
A.R.S. §§ 20-826(H), 20-934(F), 20-1057(I), 20-1342(A)(9), 20-1402(A)(5), 20-1404(G)
A.R.S. §§ 32-2841 to 32-2843

Arkansas

Ark. Stat. Ann. §§ 20-15-1301 to 20-15-1304, 26-57-201, 26-57-1101 to 26-57-1108
Ark. Stat. Ann. § 23-79-140
Ark. Stat. Ann. § 23-99-405
Ark. Stat. Ann. §§ 20-15-1001 to 20-15-1006

California

Cal Rev & Tax Code § 30461.6
Cal Health & Saf Code §§ 104875 to 104895
Cal Health & Saf Code § 1367.65
Cal Ins Code § 10123.81
Cal Wel & Inst Code § 14132.16
Cal Health & Saf Code § 1367.6
Cal Ins Code § 10123.8
Cal Wel & Inst Code § 14132.6
Cal Health & Saf Code §§ 25671(b), 25815(e), 25827, 115100, 115115
Cal Health & Saf Code §§ 1704.5, 1704.55, 109275 to 109277
Cal Rev & Tax Code §§ 18791 to 18796
Cal Health & Saf Code § 1367.635
Cal Ins Code § 10123.86
Cal Health & Saf Code §§ 104160 to 104164

Colorado

C.R.S. §§ 25-4-1501 to 25-4-1506
C.R.S. § 10-16-104(4)
C.R.S. §§ 25-11-101 to 25-11-105

Connecticut

Conn. Gen. Stat. §§ 19a-266
Conn. Gen. Stat. §§ 38a-495, 38a-503, 38a-522, 38a-530
Conn. Gen. Stat. §§ 38a-476, 38a-503a, 38a-530a
Conn. Gen. Stat. §§ 38a-469, 38a-504
Conn. Gen. Stat. §§ 12-743, 19(a)-32(b)

Delaware
>18 Del. C. § 3552
>30 Del. C. § 1159

District of Columbia
>D.C. Code §§ 35-2401 to 35-2403

Florida
>Fla. Stat. Ann. § 240.5121(4)(m)
>Fla. Stat. Ann. §§ 627.6418, 627.6419, 627.6613, 641.31095
>Fla. Stat. Ann. §§ 627.6417, 627.6515(2), 627.6612, 641.31
>Fla. Stat. Ann. § 404.22(6)
>Fla. Stat. Ann. §§ 458.324, 459.0125
>Fla. Stat. Ann. §§ 627.64171, 627.66121, 641.31
>Fla. Stat. Ann. §§ 627.64172, 627.6419, 627.6612, 641.31096

Georgia
>O.C.G.A. § 31-15-5
>O.C.G.A. § 43-34-21
>O.C.G.A. §§ 33-29-3.2, 33-30-4.2
>O.C.G.A. §§ 33-29-3.3, 33-30-4.4
>O.C.G.A. §§ 33-24-70 to 33-24-72

Hawaii
>H.R.S. §§ 431:10A-116(4), 432:1-605

Idaho
>I.C. §§ 41-2144, 41-2218, 41-3441, 41-3936, 41-4025
>I.C. § 39-3030

Illinois
>20 ILCS 2305/2, 2310/55.49
>305 ILCS 5/5-5
>215 ILCS 5/356g(a), 5/356u, 125/4-6.1
>215 ILCS 5/356g(b)
>420 ILCS 40/5, 40/24.5, 40/25, 40/28(b)
>20 ILCS 2310/55.70; 35 ILCS 5/507L, 5/509, 5/510, 1999 ILL. ALS 107
>65 ILCS 5/10-4-2.3, 105 ILCS 5/10-22.3f, 215 ILCS 5/356t, 305 ILCS 375/6.9
>625 ILCS 5/3-643

Indiana
>Burns Ind. Code Ann. §§ 20-10.1-4-13
>Burns Ind. Code Ann. §§ 27-8-14-1 to 27-8-14-6
>Burns Ind. Code Ann. §§ 27-13-7-15.3
>Burns Ind. Code Ann. § 5-10-8-7.2
>Burns Ind. Code Ann. §§ 27-8-5-26, 27-13-7-14

Iowa
>Iowa Code Ann. § 514C.4
>Iowa Code Ann. § 136C.15

Kansas

Kan. Stat. Ann. §§ 40-2229, 40-2230
Kan. Stat. Ann. § 65-2836(m)

Kentucky

KRS §§ 214.550 to 214.556
KRS §§ 304.17-316, 304.18-098, 304.32-1591, 304.38-1935
KRS §§ 304.17-3163, 304.17A-134, 304.18-0983, 304.32-1593, 304.38-1934
KRS § 311.935
KRS §§ 304.17-3165, 304.17a-135, 304.18-0985, 304.32-1595, 304.38-1936

Louisiana

La. R.S. § 17:275
La. R.S. § 46:975; 2000 La. Act 131; 2000 La. HB 153
La. R.S. § 22:215.11
1997 La. ALS 1341; 1997 La. ACT 1341; 1997 La. SB 699
La. R.S. §§ 40:1300.151 to 40:1300.154
La. R.S. § 47:120.61

Maine

24 M.R.S. §§ 2320-A, 2745-A, 2837-A, 4237-A
24 M.R.S. §§ 2332-G, 4241
24-A M.R.S. 2847-F
24 M.R.S. §§ 2320-C, 2745-C, 2837-C, 4237
24 M.R.S. § 2905A
22 M.R.S. § 8711.2

Maryland

Md. HEALTH-GENERAL Code Ann. § 20-116
Md. Ann. Code § 19-348
Md. HEALTH-GENERAL Code Ann. § 18-303
Md. Insurance Code Ann. § 15-814
Md. Insurance Code Ann. § 15-907
Md. Insurance Code Ann. § 15-815
Md. HEALTH-GENERAL Code Ann. § 19-706(d)
Md. Insurance Code Ann. § 15-832
Md. HEALTH-GENERAL Code Ann. § 20-115
Md. HEALTH-GENERAL Code Ann. § 20-113

Massachusetts

1997 Mass. ALS 43; 1997 H.B. 4700
Mass. Gen. Laws Ann. Ch. 111 § 4K
Mass. Gen. Laws Ann. Ch. 175 §§ 47G, 110; Ch. 176A § 8J; Ch. 176B § 4I;
    Ch. 176G § 4
Mass. Gen. Laws Ann. Ch. 111 § 5Q
Mass. Gen. Laws Ann. Ch. 175 § 47M; 176A § 8O; Ch. 176B § 4O; Ch. 176G § 4F;
    Ch. 32A § 17D; Ch. 175 § 47R
Mass. Gen. Laws Ann. Ch. 71 § 1

Michigan
>M.C.L. §§ 333.9501, 333.9503
>M.C.L. §§ 333.21054a, 500.3406d, 500.3616, 550.1416
>M.C.L. §§ 500.3613, 500.3406A, 550.1415
>M.C.L. §§ 333.17013, 333.17513

Minnesota
>Minn. Stat. Ann. §§ 62A.30, 62A.315, 62A.316
>Minn. Stat. Ann. § 144.651(9)
>Minn. Stat. Ann.§§ 62A.307, 62A.309

Mississippi
>Miss. Code Ann. § 83-9-108

Missouri
>R.S.Mo., § 376.782
>R.S.Mo., § 376.1209
>R.S.Mo., §§ 192.760 to 192.766
>R.S.Mo., § 376.1200

Montana
>Mont. Code Anno., §§ 33-22-132, 53-6-101(2)(c)
>Mont. Code Anno. § 33-22-135
>Mont. Code Anno. § 37-3-33
>Mont. Code Anno. § 33-22-134

Nebraska
>R.R.S. Neb. §§ 71-7617
>1999 Neb. ALS 480, 1999 Neb. Laws 480, 1999 Neb. LB 480
>R.R.S. Neb. §§ 44-785, 71-7001, 71-7002, 71-7003, 71-7012
>R.R.S. Neb. § 71-7614

Nevada
>Nev. Rev. Stat. §§ 689A.0405, 689B.0374, 695C.1735, 695B.1912
>Nev. Rev. Stat. §§ 608.157, 616.503, 617.395, 689A.041, 689B.0375, 695B.191, 695C.171
>Nev. Rev. Stat. §§ 457.182 to 457.187

New Hampshire
>N.H. RSA §§ 417-D:1 to 417-D:4
>N.H. RSA §§ 415:18-c, 420-A:13, 420-B:8e

New Jersey
>N.J. Stat. §§ 26:2-168, 45:9-22.3a, 45:9-22.3b
>N.J. Stat. § 26:2-113
>N.J. Stat. § 17B:26-2.1e, 17B:27-46.1f
>N.J. Stat. §§ 17:48-6b, 17-48a-7b, 17:48E-35, 17B:26-2-1a, 17B:27-46.1a, 26:2j-4.14
>N.J. Stat. §§ 52:9U-6.1, 54A:9-25.7, 54A:9-25.8
>N.J. Stat. §§ 17:48-6q, 17:48A-7o, 17:48E-35.14, 17B:26-2.1m, 17B:27-46.1P,
>   17B:27A-7.2, 17B:27A-19.4, 26:2J-4.15, 34:13A-30, 52:14-17.29b

New Mexico

N.M. Stat. Ann. §§ 59A-22-39, 59A-23-4, 59A-23B-3, 59A-46-41
N.M. Stat. Ann. § 27-2-12.8
N.M. Stat. Ann §§ 59A-22-39.1, 59A-46-41.1

New York

NY CLS Pub. Health §§ 2405 to 2408
NY CLS Pub. Health § 2500-c
NY CLS Ins § 4303(p)
NY CLS Ins §§ 3216(i)(20), 3221(k)(10), 4303(x)6(I)
NY CLS Pub. Health § 2404 (1-a)
NY CLS Pub. Health §§ 2410 to 2413;
NY Tax §§ 209-D, 627; NY Fin § 97-yy
NY CLS Ins. § 3224
NY CLS Educ § 804
NY CLS Pub Health §§ 2407, 2409
NY CLS St Fin § 95-a
NY Ins. Law §§ 3216(I), 3221(k), 4303(v,w)
NY CLS Pub Health § 2404(1-a)
NY CLS Veh & Tr § 404-q

North Carolina

N.C. Gen. Stat. §§ 58-50-155(a), 58-51-57, 58-65-92, 58-67-76
N.C. Gen. Stat. §§ 135-40.5(e), 135-40.6(8)(s)
N.C. Gen. Stat. §§ 58-51-62, 58-65-96, 58-67-79, 58-50-155, 135-40.6(5)
N.C. Gen. Stat. § 53-3-168

North Dakota

N.D. Cen. Code § 26.1-36-09.1

Ohio

ORC Ann. § 5.2213
ORC Ann. §§ 1742.40, 1751.62, 3923.52 to 3923.54, 5111.024

Oklahoma

63 OKL. St. §§ 1-554 to 1-558
36 OKL. St. § 6060
36 OKL. St. § 6060.5
47 OKL. St. § 1136
63 OKL. St. § 1-743

Oregon

ORS § 743.727

Pennsylvania

40 P.S. § 764c
1997 Pa. ALS 51, 1997 Pa. SB 176
35 P.S. §§ 5651 to 5664
35 P.S. §§ 5641, 5642
72 P.S. § 7315.2

Rhode Island

R.I. Gen. Laws §§ 27-18-41 to 27-18-42, 27-19-20,27-20-17, 27-41-31, 42-62-26
R.I. Gen. Laws §§ 27-18-39, 27-19-34, 27-20-21,27-20-29, 27-41-43
R.I. Gen. Laws §§ 5-37-31, 23-17-32, 27-19-21, 27-20-18, 27-41-30, 42-62-27
R.I. Gen. Laws §§ 23-67-2
R.I. Gen. Laws §§ 27-18-40, 27-19-34.1, 27-20-29.1, 27-41-43.1

South Carolina

S.C. Code Ann. § 38-71-145
S.C. Code Ann. § 38-71-130
S.C. Code Ann. § 38-71-125

South Dakota

S.D. Codified Laws §§ 34-24C-1 to 34-24C-4
S.D. Codified Laws §§ 58-17-1.1, 58-18-36, 58-38-22, 58-40-20, 58-41-35.5

Tennessee

Tenn. Code Ann. § 56-7-1012, 56-7-2502
Tenn. Code Ann. § 56-7-2507
Tenn. Code Ann. § 56-7-2504

Texas

Tex. Health & Safety Code §§ 86.001 to 86.005
Tex. Health & Safety Code §§ 86.011 to 86.012
Tex. Ins. Code art. 3.70-2(H), 3.74(3A)
Tex. Ins. Code art. 21.53D
Tex. Health & Safety Code §§ 401.421 to 401.431
Tex. Ins. Code art. 21.52G

Utah

Utah Code Ann. §§ 26-21a-101 to 26-21a-301
Utah Code Ann. §§ 19-3-103.5, 19-3-104

Vermont

8 V.S.A § 4100A
18 V.S.A § 157

Virginia

Va. Code Ann. § 38.2-3418.1
Va. Code Ann. § 2.1-20.1(B)
Va. Code Ann. § 32.1-325
Va. Code Ann. § 54.1-2971
Va. Code Ann. § 38.2-3418.1:1
Va. Code Ann. § 38.2-3418.4
Va. Code Ann. § 38.2-3418.6
2000 Va. ALS 319, 2000 Va. Acts 319, 2000 Va. Ch. 319, 2000 Va. HB 722

Washington

RCW §§ 41.05.180, 48.20.393, 48.21.225, 48.44.325, 48.46.275
RCW. §§ 48.20.395, 48.21.230, 48.44.330, 48.46.280
RCW §§ 48.20.397, 48.21.235, 48.44.335, 48.46.285

West Virginia
      W.Va. Code §§ 16-33-1 to 16-33-12
      W.Va. Code §§ 33-15-4c, 33-16-3g, 33-24-7b, 33-25-8a, 33-25A-8a
      W.Va. Code §§ 5-16-7, 5-16-9

Wisconsin
      Wis. Stat. § 255.06
      Wis. Stat. § 632.895(8)

Wyoming
      Wis. Stat. §§ 26-18-103, 26-19-107

STATUTE ABSTRACTS

What You Need To Know

Court or regulatory agency decisions may modify statutes. For example, the South Carolina Supreme Court ruled in 1987 that a health maintenance organization could not exclude coverage for post-mastectomy reconstructive surgery. In most instances, the abstracts in this digest reflect the terminology used by the respective state legislature. Statutory citations appear at the beginning of each abstract indicating the location of the law in the current edition of the appropriate state code(s). The citations do not include Act and Bill numbers, except in abstracts of laws that were not yet codified when this document was prepared. The abstracts indicate the effective dates of the statute and relevant amendments. Abstracts omit the dates of minor modifications or editorial changes found in subsequent amendments.

For statutes mandating insurance coverage for specific procedures, the abstracts indicate the types of policies subject to the mandates and any limits on coverage. The abstracts also indicate if the insurance provisions contain any quality assurance requirements.

Alabama　　　CODE OF ALA. § 22-13-6

Scope　　　Breast Cancer Screening and Education Programs

Policies and Limits　　Law provides that, as part of a program for the care and treatment of indigent cancer sufferers, females within age limits prescribed by the State Board of Health be urged to report voluntarily during "cancer detection month" for their area, to a physician of their choice, for an official examination for cancer. The examination shall include, at the Board's discretion, a diagnosis for breast cancer.

Quality Assurance　　Not indicated.

Effective Date　　1949 enactment.

Alabama   CODE OF ALA. §§ 27-50-1 TO 27-50-7

Scope   Reimbursement for Breast Cancer Screening

Women's Age,
Frequency of   40-49 Every 2 years, or more frequently upon physician's
Mammogram   recommendation

                       50+ Each year, or more frequently upon physician's
                              recommendation

Policies and Limits Law creates the state's "Breast Cancer Screening Act." In order to accomplish
                       early detection of breast cancer, Alabama law requires every health benefit plan
                       to provide coverage for screening mammography if the plan provides coverage
                       for surgical services for mastectomy.

                       Law applies to all health insurance policies (health benefit plans), which
                       includes: self-insured health plans, health maintenance organizations, preferred
                       provider organizations, medical service organizations, physician hospital
                       organizations, and all programs administered by Alabama's Medicaid Agency.

                       Law does not apply to insurance policies that are accident-only, specified
                       disease, individual hospital indemnity, credit, dental only, Medicare-supplement,
                       long-term care, disability income insurance, supplemental liability insurance,
                       workers' compensation or similar insurance, or automobile medical-payment
                       insurance.

                       Law prohibits any form of health benefit plan's attempt to penalize a physician
                       or other health care provider providing medical care consistent with this law.
                       Law imposes serious penalties upon any health care insurer that violates the
                       provisions of this code.

Quality Assurance   Not indicated.

Effective Date   October 1, 1997.

Alabama　　　　　　**2000 AL SB 559**

Scope　　　　　　　Reimbursement for Breast Reconstruction and Prosthesis

Policies and Limits　Law requires any state program funded under Title XIX of the federal Social Security Act, 42 U.S.C. Section 1396 et seq., and any other publicly funded state health care program which provides coverage for mastectomy surgery to also provide coverage for reconstruction of the breast on which surgery has been performed and surgery and reconstruction within five years of the mastectomy surgery and in the manner chosen by the patient and the physician.

　　　　　　　　　　Law defines "reconstruction."

Quality Assurance　Not indicated.

Effective Date　　　August 1, 2000

Alabama   CODE OF ALA. § 32-6-591

Scope   Special License Plates Supporting Breast Cancer Research and Education

Policies and Limits   Law provides for the distribution of state funds used to provide free mammograms to underserved women through the "Mammogram for Life Campaign."

Law provides that the additional net proceeds derived from the state's sale of distinctive "Sistas Can Survive Coalition (SCSC) motor vehicle license plates, be distributed monthly (less the cost of administration, production, and appropriation fee, taken from the first $2,000 collected in the fiscal year ending September 30, 1998) to the SCSC.

Quality Assurance   Not indicated.

Effective Date   January 1, 1998.

Alaska   ALASKA STAT. § 21.42.375

Scope   Reimbursement for Breast Cancer Screening

Woman's Age,   35-39   Baseline
Frequency
of Mammogram   40-49   Every 2 years

            50+   Each year

            Any age   If the insured has a history of breast cancer; or, upon referral by
                         a physician, if the insured's parent, or sibling has a history of
                         breast cancer.

Policies   Law requires insurers to provide coverage for low-dose mammography screening
and Limits   if the health care insurance plan covers mastectomies and prosthetic devices and
                 reconstructive surgery incident to mastectomies.

                 Law applies to any health care insurer including individual and group disability
                 insurance policies, health maintenance organizations, and hospital or medical
                 service corporation contracts.

                 The coverage for mammography *must* not be less favorable than for other
                 radiological examinations and *may* be subject to standard policy provisions (such
                 as deductible or copayment) that apply to other benefits.

                 Law does not apply to fraternal benefit societies.

                 Law defines "low-dose mammography" and "screening mammogram."

Quality Assurance   Examination must use equipment dedicated specifically for mammography.

Effective Date   September 19, 1991; last amendment effective July 1, 1997.

Arizona   **A.R.S. §§ 20-826(I), 20-934(G), 20-1057(J), 20-1342(A)(10), 20-1402(A)(6), 20-1404(H)**

Scope   Reimbursement for Breast Cancer Screening

Woman's Age,   35-39   Baseline
Frequency
of Mammogram   40-49   Every 2 years, or more frequently upon physician's
                                  recommendation

                     50+   Each year

                     Physician referral required in all cases.

Policies   Law requires health insurers to provide coverage for mammography screening if
and Limits   the policy or contract covers surgical services for mastectomies.

                     Law applies to hospital or medical service corporation contracts; benefits insurer
                     contracts; health care service organization plans; and group and blanket
                     disability contracts.

                     Law does not apply to supplemental contracts covering a specified disease or
                     other limited benefit.

Quality Assurance Mammography screening must be performed on equipment specifically dedicated
                     to mammography.

Effective Date   September 30, 1988.

Arizona   **A.R.S. §§ 20-826(H), 20-934(F), 20-1057(I), 20-1342(A)(9), 20-1402(A)(5), 20-1404(G)**

Scope   Reimbursement for Breast Reconstruction and Prosthesis

Policies
and Limits   Law requires health care plans that provide coverage for surgical services for mastectomies also provide coverage incidental to the patient's covered mastectomy for surgical services for breast reconstruction, prosthesis, treatment of physical complications for all stages of the mastectomy, and at least two external postoperative prostheses.

Law applies to hospital or medical service corporation contracts; benefits insurer contracts; health care service organization plans; and group and blanket disability contracts.

Quality Assurance   Not indicated.

Effective Date   December 31, 1981.

Arizona   **A.R.S. §§ 32-2841 to 32-2843**

Scope   Accreditation of Facilities and Technologists

Law requires that anyone who performs diagnostic or screening mammography possess a mammographic technologist certificate from the Arizona Medical Radiologic Technology Board of Examiners. The Board will issue certificates to applicants who pass an examination in mammography administered by either the Board or by the American Registry of Radiologic Technologists, complete 40 hours of didactic instruction, and 160 hours of clinical instruction taught by a facility either accredited by the American College of Radiology or licensed by the state of Arizona. Certification is valid for 2 years. Certificate renewal is available upon completion of 8 hours of continuing education in mammography, within the preceding 2 years. Temporary certificates are also available .

Law provides that physicians reading or interpreting mammographic images:

complete 40 hours of medical education credits in mammography;
be certified in diagnostic radiology by the American Board of Radiology or the American Osteopathic Board of Radiology, as applicable, or be approved by the Arizona Board of Medical Examiners or Arizona Board of Osteopathic Examiners to read or interpret mammographic images; and
have interpreted or reviewed 200 mammograms within the preceding 2 years or completed a radiology residency within the preceding 3 years; and
complete 15 hours of continuing medical education credits in mammography every 3 years and interpret or review an average of 300 mammograms per year over each 2-year period.

The Arizona Allopathic Board of Medical Examiners and the Arizona Board of Osteopathic Examiners in Medicine and Surgery shall establish minimum criteria authorizing doctors to read or interpret mammography images in lieu of certification by the American Board of Radiology or the American Osteopathic Board of Radiology. Physicians must maintain records of outcome data.

Facilities conducting patient self-referral mammographic screening examinations must submit a physician-approved guide for accepting self-referrals and a medical physicist's evaluation report of the facility to the Arizona Radiation Regulatory Agency. Facilities without on-site darkrooms must comply with special reporting requirements.

Effective Date   January 1, 1994; last amended 1999.

Arkansas **ARK. STAT. ANN. §§ 20-15-1301 TO 20-15-1304, 26-57-201,
26-57-1101 to 26-57-1108**

Scope Breast Cancer Screening and Education Programs/
Fund for Breast Cancer Research

*Policies
and Limits* Law establishes the Breast Cancer Act of 1997. Creates a breast cancer research fund and breast cancer control fund for research and services with respect to the cause, cure, detection, and prevention of breast cancer, as well as breast cancer education programs.

Law establishes a breast cancer research program within the University of Arkansas to support research into the cause, cure, treatment, earlier detection, and prevention of breast cancer. Funding of research shall be based on the research priorities established for the program and the scientific merit of the research as determined by a peer review process carried out by the Oversight Committee on Breast Cancer Research.

Law establishes a breast cancer control advisory board to recommend the allocation of funds. It establishes a breast cancer control program within the State Department of Health to provide for the early detection, diagnosis, and treatment of breast cancer. Specifically, this program shall provide for breast cancer education, awareness, and surveillance activities; breast cancer screening to include mammography; follow-up referrals and medical assistance; and, in the event of a positive diagnosis, the necessary advocacy and financial assistance to help the individual obtain treatment.

Law provides for funding through a specified tax on specified tobacco products.

Quality Assurance Not indicated.

Effective Date July 1, 1997.

Arkansas   **ARK. STAT. ANN. § 23-79-140**

Scope   Reimbursement for Breast Cancer Screening

Woman's Age,   35-40   Baseline
Frequency
of Mammogram   40-49   Every 1-2 years, based on physician's recommendation

                     50+   Each year

                     Any age   Upon physician's recommendation if the woman, her mother, or
                                    her sister has a history of breast cancer.

Policies   Law requires all health insurance providers to offer optional coverage for
and Limits   mammogram screening of breast cancer to each master group contract holder.

                     Law applies to health insurance companies, hospital service corporations, health
                     maintenance organizations, and other health insurance providers.

                     Law requires insurers to pay at least $50 for each screening mammogram,
                     including professional and technical components. For hospital outpatient
                     screening mammography, and comparable situations where the claim for
                     professional services is separate from technical services, the professional claim
                     component must be at least 40 percent of the total fee.

                     Law defines "screening mammography" and "diagnostic mammography."

Quality Assurance No insurer shall pay for mammographies performed at an unaccredited facility
                     after January 1, 1990.

Effective Date   January 1, 1990; last amendment in 1995.

Arkansas   ARK. STAT. ANN. § 23-99-405

Scope   Reimbursement for Breast Reconstruction and Prosthesis

Policies   Law requires insurers who provide benefits for mastectomy to also cover
and Limits   prosthetic devices and reconstructive surgery.

Quality Assurance   Not indicated.

Effective Date   April 8, 1997.

Arkansas   ARK. STAT. ANN. §§ 20-15-1001 to 20-15-1006

Scope   Accreditation of Facilities and Technologists

Policies   Law requires the Director of Arkansas' Department of Health, with the
and Limits   assistance of an advisory committee, to establish and to administer radiological
standards and quality assurance programs for screening and diagnostic
mammograms. The legislative intent of this law is to assure the safety and
accuracy of mammographies and to promote the highest quality imaging in the
most efficient setting to contain costs.

The Department of Health is authorized to operate a mammography standards
certificate program to issue initial and renewal certificates to mammography
facilities and to impose sanctions on facilities not meeting requirements.

The director and the committee are required to review and revise quality
standards annually, in light of current scientific knowledge, at least once every 2
years.

The Director shall establish accreditation standards for mammography facilities.
No mammography shall be performed in an unaccredited facility after January 1,
1990.

Law defines "screening mammography" and "diagnostic mammography."

Effective Date   March 2, 1995.

Arkansas　　　　ARK. STAT. ANN. § 23-99-405

Scope　　　　Reimbursement for Inpatient Treatment Following Mastectomy

Policies and Limits　　　　Laws prohibits insurers who cover mastectomy from restricting benefits for length of hospital stay in connection with a mastectomy to less than 48 hours, unless the decision to discharge the patient earlier is made by the physician in consultation with the patient.

Quality Assurance　　　　Not indicated.

Effective Date　　　　April 8, 1997.

California CAL REV & TAX CODE § 30461.6

Scope Breast Cancer Screening and Education Programs

*Policies
and Limits* Law requires that revenue from the cigarette tax increase be deposited in the State Treasury to the credit of the Breast Cancer Fund and divided equally between the Breast Cancer Research Account and the Breast Cancer Control Account.

The moneys in the Breast Cancer Research Account shall be allocated to research the cause, cure, treatment, earlier detection, and prevention of breast cancer. Of that amount, 10 percent goes to the Cancer Surveillance Section of the California Department of Health Services for the collection of breast cancer-related data and the conduct of breast cancer-related epidemiological research by the State Cancer Registry. The remaining 90 percent goes to the Breast Cancer Research Program (herein created at the University of California) for grants and contracts to researchers to research the cause, cure, treatment, prevention, and earlier detection of breast cancer.

The moneys in the Breast Cancer Control Account shall be allocated to the Breast Cancer Control Program (herein created) for early breast cancer detection services for uninsured and underinsured women. The Department of Health Services shall establish the program and administer it in accordance with P.L. 101-354.

In enacting the Breast Cancer Control Program, it is the intent of the Legislature to decrease breast cancer mortality among uninsured and underinsured women, with special emphasis on low-income, Native American, and minority women. It is the intent of the Legislature that the communities served by the program reflect the ethnic, racial, cultural, and geographic diversity of the state and that the program funds entities where uninsured and underinsured women are most likely to seek their health care.

Quality Assurance Not indicated.

Effective Date January 1, 1994.

California   CAL HEALTH & SAF CODE §§ 104875 to 104895

Scope   Breast Cancer Screening Program

Policies   Law provides for the referral of women who took diethylstilbestrol (DES) during
and Limits   pregnancy and their offspring who were exposed to diethylstilbestrol prenatally
for the purpose of follow-up care and treatment of long-term problems associated
with diethylstilbestrol exposure. Law requires the designation of at least one
program for screening and follow-up care for each health service area.

Law requires consideration of providers' compliance with state and federally
mandated standards, the location in relation to the geographic distribution of
persons exposed to diethylstilbestrol, and the capacity of the provider to properly
screen for breast cancer and any other malignancy and abnormal conditions
resulting from DES exposure.

Law requires the designation of existing facilities presently serving the
diethylstilbestrol-exposed population as screening programs pursuant to this law.
If existing positions are not available, training for screening and follow-up may
be offered to the personnel in existing facilities and clinics.

Quality Assurance   Not indicated.

Effective Date   Before 1982; last amendment in 1995.

California **CAL HEALTH & SAF CODE § 1367.65;**
CAL INS CODE § 10123.81

Scope Reimbursement for Breast Cancer Screening

Woman's Age, 35-39 Baseline
Frequency
of Mammogram 40-49 Every 2 years, or more frequently upon physician's recommendation

50+ Each year

Policies Law requires health insurers to provide coverage for mammography (upon
and Limits referral by participating nurse practitioner, certified nurse midwife, or physician) for screening or diagnostic purposes if the policy or contract covers mastectomies, and prosthetic devices, and reconstructive surgery incident to mastectomies.

Law applies to group health care service plan contracts, group disability insurance policies, self-insured employee welfare benefit plans, and Medi-Cal coverage.

Law does not establish a new mandated benefit or prevent application of deductible or copayment provisions in a policy or plan.

Quality Assurance Not indicated.

Effective Date January 1, 1988; amended 1996.

California   CAL WEL & INST CODE § 14132.16

Scope   Reimbursement for Breast Cancer Screening

Woman's Age,   Not stipulated.
Frequency
of Mammogram

Policies   Law states that Medi-Cal covers mammography for screening or diagnostic
and Limits   purposes to the extent required or permitted by federal law and upon a
                     physician's referral.

Quality Assurance Not indicated.

Effective Date   January 1, 1988.

California　　　　CAL HEALTH & SAF CODE § 1367.6;
CAL INS CODE § 10123.8;
CAL WEL & INST CODE § 14132.6

Scope　　　　Reimbursement for Breast Reconstruction and Prosthesis

Policies　　　Law requires that health insurers covering surgical services for mastectomies
and Limits　　also provide coverage for prosthetic devices or reconstructive surgery incident to
　　　　　　　the mastectomy.

　　　　　　　Law applies to group health care service plan contracts, group disability
　　　　　　　insurance policies, self-insured employee welfare benefit plans, and Medi-Cal
　　　　　　　coverage.

　　　　　　　Coverage is subject to deductible or coinsurance provisions and all other terms
　　　　　　　and conditions applicable to benefits.

Quality Assurance　　Not indicated.

Effective Date　　July 1, 1980; amended 1996.

California   CAL HEALTH & SAF CODE §§ 25671(b), 25815(e), 25827, 115100, 115115

Scope   Accreditation of Facilities and Technologists

Policies   Law requires that anyone performing mammography have a current and valid
and Limits   certificate in mammographic radiologic technology.

                     Law requires registration and certification of all mammography equipment by the
                     California Department of Health Services. All X-ray machines used for
                     mammography must be specifically designed for mammography and be inspected
                     by the Department or certified by the American College of Radiology
                     Mammography Accreditation Program or an equivalent program.

                     The person registering X-ray equipment must obtain and maintain a
                     Mammography Quality Assurance Program to include a Mammography Quality
                     Assurance Manual for the identification of mammography quality assurance tests
                     performed, test frequency, test equipment used, maintenance and calibration of
                     test equipment, and qualifications of individuals who perform the tests in order to
                     ensure compliance with the May 1990 version of "Rules of Good Practice for
                     Supervision and Operation of Mammographic X-Ray Equipment" or health
                     department regulations.

                     All persons who have a certificate for mammography equipment must follow the
                     Department's quality assurance program. Quality assurance tests must be
                     performed on mobile vans or units after each relocation.

Effective Date   July 15, 1993.

California   CAL HEALTH & SAF CODE §§ 1704.5, 1704.55,
                  109275 TO 109277

Scope   Alternative Therapies/Breast Cancer Screening and Education Programs

Policies   Law states that unprofessional conduct includes the failure of a physician to
and Limits   inform a patient being treated for any form of breast cancer of alternative,
                  efficacious methods of treatment specified in the standardized written summary
                  developed by the Department on recommendation of the Cancer Advisory
                  Council.

                  Law requires health facilities and licensed physicians or surgeons, who rent or
                  own the premises where their practice is located, to post a sign with the following
                  information in an area that is proximate to where breast cancer screening or
                  biopsy procedures are performed:

                  "BE INFORMED" " If you are a patient being treated for any form of breast
                  cancer, or prior to performance of a biopsy for breast cancer, your physician or
                  surgeon is required to provide you with a written summary of alternative
                  efficacious methods of treatment, pursuant to Section 109275 of the California
                  Health and Safety Code. "The information about methods of treatment was
                  developed by the State Department of Health Services to inform patients of the
                  advantages, disadvantages, risks, and descriptions of procedures."

                  Signs must be posted in English, Spanish, and Chinese.

Quality Assurance Not indicated.

Effective Date   1980 enactment; amended September 29, 1996.

California   CAL REV & TAX CODE §§ 18791 to 18796

Scope   Income Tax Checkoff for Breast Cancer Research

Policies   Law creates the California Breast Cancer Research Fund and provides that
and Limits   individuals may designate on tax returns that a contribution in excess of tax
                  liability be made to the Fund.

                  Law directs the California Franchise Tax Board to revise return forms to include
                  a space labeled "California Breast Cancer Research Fund."

                  Funds shall be allocated as follows:

                  #   to the Franchise Tax Board and the Controller for the reimbursement of
                             all costs incurred by them; and

                  #   to the University of California for the support of the Breast Cancer
                             Research Program for purposes solely related to breast cancer research
                             as stated in Section 104145 of Chapter 2 of Part 1 of Division 103 of the
                             Health and Safety Code (see Breast Cancer Research Programs, below).

                  Provision shall remain in effect until January 1, 2003.

Quality Assurance   Not indicated.

Effective Date   January 1, 1994; amended January 1, 1998.

California   CAL HEALTH & SAF CODE § 1367.635
                   CAL INS CODE § 10123.86

Scope   Reimbursement for Length of Stay/Inpatient Care Following Mastectomy

Policies   Law prohibits health insurers that provide coverage for breast cancer treatment
and Limits   from limiting inpatient hospital coverage for surgical procedures known as
                   mastectomies and lymph node dissections to any period that is less than that
                   determined by the attending physician and surgeon to be medically necessary, in
                   accordance with sound clinical principles and processes, and in consultation with
                   the insured patient.

                   Law also requires insurers that provide coverage for mastectomies to provide
                   coverage for all complications from a mastectomy, including lymphedema.

                   Insurance plans may not deny an insured individual for the purpose of avoiding
                   the above requirements, provide monetary incentives for accepting less than these
                   requirements, penalize health care providers for providing care in accordance
                   with these requirements, or provide incentives to a provider to provide less than
                   the required care mandated by this law. In addition, insurers may not restrict
                   benefits for any portion of a hospital stay in a manner that is less favorable than
                   the benefits provided for any preceding portion of the stay.

                   Law does not require patients to have the mastectomy in a hospital or stay in the
                   hospital for a fixed period of time following the procedure.

                   Law applies to all health care service plan contracts and disability insurance
                   policies.

                   Law defines the following terms: coverage for prosthetic devices or
                   reconstructive surgery, prosthetic devices, mastectomy, and symmetry.

Quality Assurance Not indicated.

Effective Date   July 1, 1999

California   CAL HEALTH & SAF CODE §§ 104160 to 104164

Scope   Breast Cancer Treatment Program

Policies   Law describes the award of a contract to provide breast cancer treatment to
and Limits   uninsured and underinsured women with incomes at or below 200 percent of the
          federal poverty level.

          Law requires contract bidder to be a nonprofit organization established under
          Section 501(c)(3) of the federal Internal Revenue Code. Law lists additional
          eligibility criteria that organizations must possess in order to bid for the contract.

          Law states that breast cancer treatment includes, but shall not be limited to,
          lumpectomy, mastectomy, chemotherapy, hormone therapy, radiotherapy,
          reconstructive surgery, and breast implant surgery.

          Law states that the department shall contract for breast cancer treatment services
          only during a fiscal year in which the Legislature has appropriated funds to the
          department for this purpose.

Quality Assurance   Not indicated.

Effective Date   July 22, 1999, operative until July 1, 2000 (repealed as of that date, unless a
          later enacted statute is enacted before July 1, 2000, deletes or extends that date)

Colorado   **C.R.S. 25-4-1501 to 25-4-1506**

Scope   Breast Cancer Screening and Education Programs

Policies   Law establishes a breast cancer screening fund to improve the availability of
and Limits   breast cancer screening. The fund shall be used to create and develop a breast
                      cancer screening program, operated either by private contract or by the Colorado
                      Department of Public Health and Environment, and to create and operate a
                      referral service for the benefit of women for whom further treatment is indicated
                      by the breast cancer screening.

                      Law directs the executive director of the Department to appoint an advisory
                      board to recommend guidelines for the program services, and necessary rules and
                      regulations.

Quality Assurance   Not indicated.

Effective Date   April 7, 1988.

Colorado   **C.R.S. 10-16-104(4)**

Scope   Reimbursement for Breast Cancer Screening

Woman's Age,   35-39   Baseline
Frequency
of Mammogram   40-49   Every 2 years, but at least once a year for women with risk
                                   factors as determined by a physician

                     50-65   Each year

Policies   Law requires that insurers provide coverage for routine or diagnostic screening
and Limits   by low-dose mammography for the presence of breast cancer in adult women.

                     Law applies to all individual and group sickness and accident insurance policies,
                     except supplemental policies covering a specified disease or other limited benefit,
                     plus all individual and group health care service or indemnity contracts and any
                     other group health care coverage provided to state residents.

                     This benefit does not diminish or limit other diagnostic benefits under any policy.

                     Coverage shall be the *lesser of* $60 or the actual cost of the screening. The
                     minimum benefit shall be adjusted according to the Consumer Price Index.

                     Law defines "low-dose mammography."

Quality Assurance Examination must use equipment dedicated specifically for mammography.

Effective Date   July 1, 1992; last amendment effective May 16, 1995.

Colorado   **C.R.S. §§ 25-11-101 to 25-11-105**

Scope   Accreditation of Facilities and Technologists

Policies   Law provides that the mammography quality assurance advisory committee
and Limits   established by the Colorado Women's Cancer Control Initiative in the Colorado
                             Department of Public Health and Environment review the provision of
                             mammography services and make recommendations to the State Board of Health
                             concerning quality assurance, including recommendations on the implementation
                             of the Mammography Quality Standards Act of 1992.

                             Law directs that regulations provide that mammographers must obtain training
                             and education through an organization specified by the Board of Health.
                             Mammographers must have achieved a passing score for the limited scope of
                             practice in radiology as administered by the American Registry of Radiological
                             Technologists or similar instruction. All regulations shall be modeled after the
                             Mammography Quality Standards Act of 1992 and those regulations proposed
                             by the Conference of Radiation Control Program Directors, Inc.

                             No person shall perform a mammography exam without being approved by the
                             Department as meeting the qualifications adopted by the Board of Health.

Effective Date   July 1, 1993; provisions in the first paragraph above (C.R.S. 25-11-105)
                             repealed effective July 1, 1998.

Connecticut   CONN. GEN. STAT. § 19a-266

Scope   Breast Cancer Screening and Education Programs

Policies   Law establishes a breast and cervical cancer early detection and treatment referral
and Limits   program within the Department of Public Health. The program is to promote
                     screening, detection, and treatment of breast cancer and cervical cancer among
                     unserved or underserved populations; to educate the public regarding breast
                     cancer and the benefits of early detection; and to provide counseling and referral
                     services for treatment.

                     The Department of Public Health must provide unserved and underserved
                     populations, within existing appropriations and through contracts with health care
                     providers: (i) one mammogram each year for ages 45 to 64; and
                     (ii) one mammogram each year for ages 35 to 44 with a first degree female
                     relative who has had breast cancer or other risk factors of equal weight.

                     The program shall establish a public education and outreach initiative; develop
                     professional education programs; and establish a tracking and follow-up system
                     for women screened under the program.

                     The Department may accept funds from federal, other public, or private sources
                     to support the program.

Quality Assurance The program shall ensure that participating providers are in compliance with
                     national and state quality assurance legislative mandates.

Effective Date   July 1, 1996.

Connecticut   CONN. GEN. STAT. §§ 38a-495, 38a-503, 38a-522, 38a-530

Scope	Reimbursement for Breast Cancer Screening	
Woman's Age,	35-39	Baseline
Frequency		
of Mammogram	40-49	Every 2 years, or more frequently upon physician's recommendation
	50+	Each year

Policies Law requires all medicare supplement insurance policies provide for
and Limits mammographic examinations each year, or more frequently upon physician's
recommendation, when such examinations are not paid for by Medicare.

Law applies to any individual or group health insurance policy delivered or
issued for delivery to any resident of the state of Connecticut who is eligible for
Medicare.

Breast cancer screening benefits are subject to any policy provisions which apply
to other services covered by the policy.

Quality Assurance Not indicated.

Effective Date October 1, 1988; last amended in 1992 to make provisions of the section
applicable to Medicare supplement policy regulations adopted pursuant to Sec.
38(a)-495(a).

Connecticut CONN. GEN. STAT. §§ 38a-476, 38a-503a, 38a-530a

Scope Restrictions on Denial of Insurance Coverage for Breast Cancer Survivors

Policies and Limits Law states that no individual or group health insurance plan or insurance arrangement may refuse to cover an applicant due to a history of breast cancer if the applicant has remained free from breast cancer for at least 5 years prior to the applicant's request for coverage. Routine follow-up care to determine whether breast cancer has reoccurred in a person who has been previously determined to be breast cancer free shall not be considered a circumstance for denial of insurance *unless* evidence of breast cancer is newly found during or as a result of such follow-up. Additionally, generic information shall not be treated as a circumstance for denial of insurance in the absence of a diagnosis of the condition related to such information. Pregnancy shall not be considered a preexisting condition.

The insurance carrier may require that the applicant submit to a physical examination.

Quality Assurance Not indicated.

Effective Date October 1, 1996.

Connecticut   CONN. GEN. STAT. § 38a-469, 38a-504

Scope   Reimbursement for Breast Reconstruction and Prosthesis

Policies   Connecticut law requires all individual health insurance policies provide
and Limits   coverage for breast reconstruction and prosthesis following the surgical removal
                     of tumors.

                     Law applies to all insurance companies, hospital service corporations, medical
                     service corporations, health care centers, or fraternal benefit societies.

                     For the surgical removal of breasts due to the surgical removal of tumors, the
                     required coverage must provide at least a yearly benefit of $500 for
                     reconstructive surgery and at least $300 yearly benefit for prosthesis, for each
                     breast removal.

                     For mastectomy, the required coverage must provide benefits for "the reasonable
                     costs of reconstructive surgery on each breast on which a mastectomy has been
                     performed, and on a nondiseased breast to produce a symmetrical appearance."

                     Such required benefits are subject to the same terms and conditions applicable to
                     all other benefits under the respective policy.

                     Law defines "reconstructive surgery" and "health insurance policy."

Quality Assurance Not indicated.

Effective Date   1991. (Law applicable to breast reconstruction after mastectomy, effective July
                     1, 1997.)

Connecticut   CONN. GEN. STAT. §§ 12-743, 19(A)-32(B)

Scope   Income Tax Checkoff for Breast Cancer Funds

Policies   This law establishes a separate breast cancer research and education account
and Limits   within the General Fund. Directs the Commissioner of Revenue services to revise
                        the tax return form to allow taxpayers to indicate a donation to the account when
                        filing their returns, and to promote the income tax contribution system and the
                        breast cancer research and education account. Money deposited in this account
                        shall be used by the Department of Public Health to assist breast cancer research,
                        education, and community service programs.

Quality Assurance   Not indicated.

Effective Date   June 26, 1997, and applicable to taxable years commencing on or after January
                        1, 1997.

Delaware   **18 DEL. C. § 3552**

Scope	Reimbursement for Breast Cancer Screening

Woman's Age, *Frequency* *of Mammogram*	35 (at least)	Baseline (for asymptomatic women), or as the Director of the Division of Public Health shall otherwise declare appropriate
	40-50	Every 1-2 years but no sooner than 2 years after a woman's baseline mammogram (for asymptomatic women), or as otherwise declared appropriate by the woman's attending physician or Director of the Division of Public Health.
	50+	Each year (for asymptomatic women), or as the Director of the Division of Public Health shall otherwise declare appropriate
	Any age	When prescribed by a physician based on an evaluation of physical conditions, symptoms, or risk factors which indicates a breast cancer pathological probability higher than that of the general population.

Policies *and Limits*	Law requires that all group and blanket health insurance, providing benefits for outpatient services also provide benefits for periodic mammographic examinations, notwithstanding policy exclusions for services which are part of annual or routine examinations.

Law applies to any health insurer and health service corporation.

The benefit paid shall not exceed the least expensive cost of a mammogram at a qualified imaging facility located at a fixed location in the Delaware county the woman resides, is principally employed, the location of the employers under whose group or blanket health plan the woman is covered, or, in which the woman actually has the mammogram. The benefit cost shall include both the facility and the radiologist's fees.

Law defines "qualified imaging facility."

Quality Assurance	Not indicated.

Effective Date	Last amendment effective July 13, 1998.

Delaware   **30 DEL. C. § 1159**

Scope   Income Tax Checkoff for Breast Cancer Education and Early Detection

Policies   Law establishes the Breast Cancer Education and Early Detection Fund.
and Limits   Taxpayers can designate contributions of one dollar or more to the Fund on their
                  state income tax returns. Contributions do not reduce the amount of taxes owed;
                  taxpayers can enclose their contribution with any taxes owed or direct that it be
                  deducted from their tax refund.

                  The Division of Revenue shall forward all contributions to Women and Wellness,
                  Inc., which shall deposit them to the credit of the Delaware chapter of the
                  National Breast Cancer Coalition to be used for breast cancer education and
                  early detection.

                  Women and Wellness, Inc. shall submit reports on revenues, expenditures, and
                  activities as requested to the Delaware State Clearinghouse Committee.

Quality Assurance   Not indicated.

Effective Date   July 9, 1996; former Del. Code Ann. 30 § 1158, redesignated as § 1159 in 1997.

District of Columbia

D.C. CODE §§ 35-2401 to 35-2403

Scope Reimbursement for Breast Cancer Screening

Woman's Age, Frequency of Mammogram Age not stipulated.

Policies and Limits Law provides for a baseline mammogram and an annual screening mammogram.

Law applies to any individual or group health insurance policy or service, including Medicaid, offered by Group Hospitalization and Medical Services, Inc., a health insurance company, a health self-insured, an insurance purchasing trust, or any health maintenance organization.

Law does not apply to hospital indemnity policies, disability insurance policies, accident only policies, or student accident policies.

Law defines "baseline mammogram" and "screening mammogram."

Quality Assurance Not indicated.

Effective Date One hundred twenty days after March 7, 1991.

Florida **FLA. STAT. ANN. § 240.5121(4)(m)**

Scope Breast Cancer Screening and Education Programs

Policies Law directs Florida Cancer Control and Research Advisory Council to develop
and Limits and implement an educational program to inform citizen groups, associations,
and voluntary organizations about early detection and treatment of breast cancer.

If funds are specifically appropriated by the legislature, the Council shall develop
or purchase and periodically update a standardized written summary of the
medically viable treatment alternatives for breast cancer. This information will be
made available to physicians and surgeons for their use in accordance with
sections 458.324 and 459.0125 (see Alternative Therapies, below).

Quality Assurance Not indicated.

Effective Date July 1, 1995.

Florida   FLA. STAT. ANN. §§ 627.6418, 627.6419, 627.6613, 641.31095

Scope   Reimbursement for Breast Cancer Screening

Woman's Age,   35-39   Baseline
Frequency
of Mammogram   40-49   Every 2 years, or more frequently upon physician's

   50+   Each year

   Any age   One or more mammograms each year, based on a physician's recommendation, for any woman who is at risk for breast cancer because of a personal or family history of breast cancer, because she has not given birth before the age of 30, or because she has a history of biopsy-proven benign breast disease.

Policies   Law applies to accident or health insurance policies and health maintenance
and Limits   contracts, but does not apply to disability income, specified disease, or hospital indemnity policies. Law does not require a physician's referral.

   Coverage is subject to deductibles and coinsurance provisions that apply to outpatient visits and terms and conditions applicable to other benefits. However, insurers must make available, for an appropriate additional premium, identical coverage that is not subject to deductibles or coinsurance.

   Insurers may not refuse to issue or renew a policy or contract, and may not cancel or exclude benefits from a policy or contract, solely because the insured has been diagnosed as having a fibrocystic condition or a nonmalignant lesion that demonstrates a predisposition, unless the condition is diagnosed through a breast biopsy that demonstrates an increased disposition to developing breast cancer.

Quality Assurance   Coverage applies to mammograms obtained in an office, facility, or health testing service registered with the Florida Department of Health and Rehabilitative Services for breast cancer screening.

   Law does not affect requirements or prohibitions on who may perform, analyze, or interpret a mammogram or the person to whom the results may be furnished or released.

Effective Date   Amended July 1, 1995.

Florida　　　　　FLA. STAT. ANN. §§ 627.6417, 627.6515(2), 627.6612, 641.31

Scope　　　　　Reimbursement for Breast Reconstruction and Prosthesis

Policies　　　Law requires that accident and health insurance policies, and group, blanket, or
and Limits　　franchise accident or health insurance policies that cover mastectomies also
　　　　　　　　provide, as part of the application, coverage for prosthetic devices and breast
　　　　　　　　reconstructive surgery incident to mastectomy. Breast reconstructive surgery
　　　　　　　　must be performed in a manner chosen by the treating physician, consistent with
　　　　　　　　prevailing medical standards, and in consultation with the patient.

　　　　　　　　Law does not apply to disability income, specified disease, or hospital indemnity
　　　　　　　　policies.

　　　　　　　　Law allows the insurer to charge an appropriate additional premium for such
　　　　　　　　coverage. Coverage is subject to deductibles or coinsurance provisions and all
　　　　　　　　other terms and conditions applicable to benefits.

　　　　　　　　Law defines "mastectomy" and "breast reconstructive surgery."

Quality Assurance　Not indicated.

Effective Date　July 2, 1987; last amended October 1, 1997.

Florida   **FLA. STAT. ANN. § 404.22(6)**

Scope   Accreditation of Facilities

Policies   Law requires that all radiation machines used for mammography meet the
and Limits   accreditation criteria of the American College of Radiology or similar criteria
                           established by the Florida Department of Health and Rehabilitative Services.

                           Law requires that all radiation machines used for mammography be specifically
                           designed for mammography and be used exclusively for mammography.

                           Law defines mammography.

Effective Date   October 1, 1991.

Florida FLA. STAT. ANN. §§ 458.324, 459.0125

Scope Alternative Therapies

Policies
and Limits Law directs physicians treating patients at high risk of being diagnosed for breast cancer to: inform those patients of the medically viable treatment alternatives available; describe such treatment alternatives; and explain the relative advantages, disadvantages, and risks associated with the treatment alternatives to the extent deemed necessary to allow the patient to make a prudent decision regarding such treatment options.

Quality Assurance Not indicated.

Effective Date 1984 enactment.

Florida   FLA. STAT. ANN. §§ 627.64171, 627.66121, 641.31

Scope   Reimbursement for Length of Stay and Outpatient Care Following Mastectomy

Policies   Law prohibits insurers that provide coverage for breast cancer treatment
and Limits   from limiting inpatient hospital coverage for mastectomy to any period that is
                 less than that determined by the treating physician to be medically necessary, in
                 accordance with prevailing medical standards, and in consultation with the
                 insured patient.

                 Law also requires insurers that provide coverage for mastectomies to provide
                 coverage for outpatient post-surgical follow-up care in keeping with prevailing
                 medical standards, by a licensed health care professional qualified to provide this
                 care. The physician, in consultation with the patient, shall determine the best
                 setting for this outpatient care.

                 Insurance plans may not deny an insured individual for the purpose of avoiding
                 the above requirements, provide monetary incentives for accepting less than these
                 requirements, penalize health care providers for providing care in accordance
                 with these requirements, or provide incentives to a provider to provide less than
                 the required care mandated by this law. In addition, insurers may not restrict
                 benefits for any portion of a hospital stay in a manner that is less favorable than
                 the benefits provided for any preceding portion of the stay.

                 Law does not require patients to have the mastectomy in a hospital or stay in the
                 hospital for a fixed period of time following the procedure. Law permits insurers
                 to impose deductibles, coinsurance, and other policies that are consistent with
                 those imposed for other benefits.

                 Law does not apply to disability income, specified disease (other than cancer), or
                 hospital indemnity policies.

                 Law defines "mastectomy."

Quality Assurance   Not indicated.

Effective Date   October 1, 1997.

Florida　　　　　　**FLA. STAT. ANN. §§ 627.64172, 627.6419, 627.6612, 641.31096**

Scope　　　　　　Restrictions on Denial of Insurance Coverage for Breast Cancer Survivors

Policies　　　　　Law states that routine follow-up care to determine whether breast cancer has
and Limits　　　　reoccurred in a person who has been previously determined to be free of the
　　　　　　　　　disease shall not be seen as constituting medical advice, diagnosis, care, or
　　　　　　　　　treatment for purposes of determining preexisting conditions, unless evidence of
　　　　　　　　　breast cancer is found during or as a result of this follow-up care.

　　　　　　　　　In addition, an insurer may not deny the issuance or renewal of insurance
　　　　　　　　　coverage because an insured person has been diagnosed as having a fibrocystic
　　　　　　　　　condition or other nonmalignant lesion that demonstrates a predisposition to
　　　　　　　　　breast cancer, unless the condition is diagnosed through a breast biopsy. The law
　　　　　　　　　also states that an insurer may not deny coverage to breast cancer survivors
　　　　　　　　　solely due to a history of breast cancer if the person has been free from the
　　　　　　　　　disease for more than 2 years before their request for coverage.

Quality Assurance　Not indicated.

Effective Date　　October 1, 1997.

Georgia **O.C.G.A. § 31-15-5**

Scope Breast Cancer Screening and Education Programs

Policies Law requires the Commissioner of Health, with the advice of the Cancer
and Limits Advisory Committee, to:

Develop standards for determining eligibility of patients for care and treatment
under the program.

Allocate state matching funds.

Extend financial aid to cancer patients.

Assist in the development and execution of programs for the early detection of
cancer, including mammography screening for breast cancer.

Institute and support, directly or through health organizations such as the
American Cancer Society and the Georgia Cancer Management Network,
educational programs for physicians, providers of health care, and the public
concerning cancer, including the dissemination of information regarding
prevention, early detection, and treatment.

Support a statewide cancer registry.

Effective Date 1977

Georgia   **O.C.G.A. § 43-34-21**

Scope   Breast Cancer Screening and Education Programs

Policies   Law transfers from the Secretary of the state of Georgia to its newly created
and Limits   board established to be known as the Composite State Board of Medical
                      Examiners (the "board") jurisdiction relative to the protection of the public health
                      and regulation of the practice of medicine.

                      Law requires that when funds are specifically appropriated for such purpose, the
                      board must publish an informational booklet on breast cancer and its treatment;
                      and, make it available to all appropriate physicians in the state urging each
                      physician to distribute a copy of the booklet to every breast cancer patient.
                      Copies of the booklet are also to be made available to all other persons upon
                      request and at a fee (sufficient to cover costs of printing and distribution). The
                      booklet is to be updated and redistributed at such times as the board deems
                      necessary.

                      The booklet must contain a summary of the latest information on breast cancer
                      and discuss generally accepted, widely prevailing, medical and surgical
                      treatments for breast cancer. The booklet must also include a valid assessment of
                      the relative risks and benefits of such treatment methods.

Quality Assurance   Not indicated.

Effective Date   Last amendment effective July 1, 1999.

Georgia   **O.C.G.A. §§ 33-29-3.2, 33-30-4.2**

Scope   Reimbursement for Breast Cancer Screening

Woman's Age,   35-39   Baseline
Frequency
of Mammogram   40-49   Once every 2 years

                    50+   Once each year

                    Any age   When ordered by a physician for a "female at risk" (a woman
                                   who has: a personal history of breast cancer; biopsy-proven
                                   benign breast disease; a grandmother, mother, sister, or daughter
                                   with a history of breast cancer; not given birth by age 30).

Policies   Law requires insurers in the state of Georgia, who issue any woman an
and Limits   individual or group accident and sickness insurance policy shall include in each
                    such policy coverage for mammography screening.

                    Law applies to individual accident and sickness insurance policies issued by
                    fraternal benefit societies, nonprofit hospital service corporations, nonprofit
                    medical service corporations, health care plans, health maintenance
                    organizations, and similar other entities.

                    The mammography screening coverage required by the law *may* be subject to
                    such exclusions, reductions, coverage limitations, deductibles, or coinsurance
                    provision(s) as may be approved by the Commissioner.

                    Nothing in the law prohibits policies from providing benefits or mammogram
                    testing frequencies greater than those required by law.

                    Law defines "mammogram."

Quality Assurance Mammography must use equipment approved by the Georgia Department of
                     Health and Human Resources. The equipment must be dedicated specifically for
                     mammography.

                     Coverage shall include a physician's or experienced radiologist's interpretation of
                     the results in accordance with American College of Radiology guidelines.

Effective Date   July 1, 1992.

Georgia   **O.C.G.A. §§ 33-29-3.3, 33-30-4.4**

Scope　　　　　　　Reimbursement for Bone Marrow Transplant for Breast Cancer

Policies　　　　　Law requires that all insurers who issue, deliver, issue for delivery, or renew
and Limits　　　individual or group major medical accident and sickness insurance make
　　　　　　　　　coverage available for bone marrow transplants for the treatment of breast
　　　　　　　　　cancer.

　　　　　　　　　Insurers include: fraternal benefit societies, nonprofit hospital service
　　　　　　　　　corporations, nonprofit medical service corporations, health care plans, health
　　　　　　　　　maintenance organizations, or similar entities.

　　　　　　　　　Such optional coverage must be at least as extensive and provide at least the
　　　　　　　　　same degree of coverage provided by the respective policy for the treatment of
　　　　　　　　　other types of physical illnesses. Additionally, such optional coverage must be
　　　　　　　　　made available to the insured's spouse and dependents if they are otherwise
　　　　　　　　　covered under the respective policy.

　　　　　　　　　Any exclusion, reduction, or limitation on coverage, deductible, or coinsurance
　　　　　　　　　provision to the optional coverage required by law must apply generally to other
　　　　　　　　　similar benefits under the policy. Law does not prohibit policies from offering
　　　　　　　　　benefits greater than those required by law. Nor does the law prohibit inclusion
　　　　　　　　　of coverage for bone marrow transplants, different from the coverage provided in
　　　　　　　　　the same policy for physical illness if the policy holder chooses not to purchase
　　　　　　　　　the optional coverage which the law requires be made available.

Quality Assurance　Not indicated.

Effective Date　　July 1, 1995; no subsequent amendments.

Georgia   **O.C.G.A. §§ 33-24-70 to 33-24-72**

Scope   Reimbursement for Length of Stay/Inpatient Care Following Mastectomy

Policies   Law prohibits health insurers that provide coverage for breast cancer treatment
and Limits   from limiting inpatient hospital coverage for surgical procedures known as
mastectomies and lymph node dissections to any period that is less than that
determined by the attending physician and surgeon to be medically necessary, in
accordance with sound clinical principles and processes, and in consultation with
the insured patient.

Law also requires insurers that provide coverage for mastectomies to provide
coverage for outpatient post-surgical follow-up care by a physician, a
physician's assistant, or a registered professional nurse with experience and
training in postsurgical care.

Insurance plans may not deny an insured individual for the purpose of avoiding
the above requirements, provide monetary incentives for accepting less than these
requirements, penalize health care providers for providing care in accordance
with these requirements, or provide incentives to a provider to provide less than
the required care mandated by this law.

Law finds and declares that there is sufficient scientific data to question the
safety and appropriateness of making mastectomies and lymph node dissections
outpatient procedures.

Law requires insurers to provide notice, in writing, to policyholders regarding the
coverage.

Law applies to all individual and group sickness and accident insurance policies,
except supplemental policies covering a specified disease or other limited benefit,
plus all individual and group health care service or indemnity contracts and any
other group health care coverage provided to state residents.

Law defines the following terms: attending physician, health benefit policy,
insurer, lymph node dissection, and mastectomy.

Quality Assurance   Not indicated.

Effective Date   July 1, 1999.

Hawaii   **H.R.S. §§ 431:10A-116(4), 432:1-605**

Scope   Reimbursement for Breast Cancer Screening

Woman's Age,   40+   Once every year
Frequency
of Mammogram   Any age   Upon recommendation of insured's physician if the insured, her
                 mother, or her sister, has a history of breast cancer.

Policies   Law requires insurers to provide coverage for low-dose screening mammography
and Limits   for yet undetected breast cancers.

            Law applies to every accident and sickness insurance policy delivered or issued
            for delivery in the state of Hawaii.

            Law does *not* include coverage under insurance policies that provide only
            coverage for specified diseases or other limited benefits.

            Services provided are subject to any applicable coinsurance provisions in force
            under the respective policy.

            Law defines "low-dose mammography."

Quality Assurance   Law requires the Director of Health to monitor the availability of safe equipment
            and trained personnel and to modify the age and frequency guidelines if
            warranted to assure that the demand for screening does not exceed the ability of
            the medical community to safely provide the services.

Effective Date   1987; last amendment effective April 15, 1999.

Idaho   **I.C. §§ 41-2144, 41-2218, 41-3441, 41-3926, 41-4025**

Scope   Reimbursement for Breast Cancer Screening

Woman's Age,   35-39   Baseline
Frequency of
Mammogram   40-49   Every 2 years, or more frequently upon recommendation of
          insured's physician

          50+   Once each year

          Any age   For any woman desiring a mammogram for "medical cause"
          (coverage shall not exceed the cost of the examination)

Policies   Law requires all health insurance policies that cover mastectomies to provide
and Limits   minimum mammography examination or equivalent examination coverage.

          Law applies to individual, group, and blanket disability insurance policies; self-
          funded health care plans; hospital and professional service corporations; health
          maintenance organizations; and managed care plans.

          Law does *not* apply to health insurance policies that cover only specific accidents
          or disease, hospital indemnity, Medicare supplement, long-term care, or other
          such limited benefit health insurance policies.

          Law defines "mastectomy."

Quality Assurance   Not indicated.

Effective Date   July 1, 1992; amended July 1, 1997.

Idaho **I.C. § 39-3030**

Scope Accreditation of Facilities

Policies Law requires registration with the Idaho Department Health and Welfare (the
and Limits "department") of all radiation machines used to perform mammography.

Such machines *must* meet current criteria established and published by the
American College of Radiology Mammography Accreditation Program; or an
equivalent standard adopted by the department. The department may withdraw
mammography authorization for machines that do not meet the college's program
standards.

Law defines "radiation machine" and "mammography system."

Effective Date January 1, 1993.

Illinois   **20 ILCS 2305/2, 2310/55.49**

Scope   Breast Cancer Screening and Education Programs

Policies   Law requires that the Illinois Department of Public Health publish, in layman's
and Limits   language, a standardized written summary outlining the methods for the early
          detection and diagnosis of breast cancer.

          By law, the summary must:

          # contain a panorama of guidelines recommended for the early detection and
          diagnosis of breast cancer.

          # advise women to seek mammography service from federally certified facilities
          only.

          # contain medically viable alternative treatment methods.

          # provide information about breast reconstruction.

          # provide the advantages, disadvantages, risks, and dangers of the various
          treatment and reconstruction methods.

          The Department shall additionally: (i) publish a Spanish translation of the
          summary; (ii) conduct public information campaigns in order to distribute the
          summary to Illinois's Hispanic women population; (iii) provide the summary for
          public distribution to hospitals, public health centers, appropriate physicians for
          public dissemination, and to all other interested persons upon request.

          The Department's update of the summary shall be done whenever necessary, but
          under no circumstance, less than once every two years.

          The Department shall consult with the Advisory Board of Cancer Control, the
          Illinois State Medical Society, and consumer groups.

Quality Assurance   Not indicated.

Effective Date   July 1, 1989.

Illinois   **305 ILCS 5/5-5**

Scope   Reimbursement for Breast Cancer Screening

Woman's Age,   35-39   Baseline
Frequency of
Mammogram   40+   Once every year.

Policies   Law authorizes the Illinois Department to provide and pay for low-dose
and Limits   mammography screening for the presence of yet undetected or diagnosed breast
                   cancer in women eligible under this law for medical assistance.

                   All screenings *must* include a physical breast exam, instruction on how and how
                   frequently to perform self-examination.

                   Law defines "low-dose mammography."

Quality Assurance   The examination must use equipment dedicated specifically for mammography.

Effective Date   January 1, 1991; last amendment effective December 22, 1999.

Illinois   **215 ILCS 5/356g(a), 5/356u, 125/4-6.1**

Scope   Reimbursement for Breast Cancer Screening

Woman's Age,   35-39   Baseline
Frequency
of Mammogram   40+   Once every year

Policies   Law requires every group and individual insurance policy provide, within the
and Limits   provisions of the respective policy, coverage for low-dose screening
                    mammography for the presence of yet undetected or undiagnosed breast cancer.

                    Law applies to every group or individual insurance policy, contract, or certificate
                    of insurance; every contract evidence of coverage issued by health maintenance
                    organizations; the Illinois Department of Public Aid (for those eligible for
                    medical assistance); and self-insured counties providing coverage for their
                    employees (provided that state funds are appropriated for reimbursement).

                    Law requires that the mammography benefits be at least as favorable as for other
                    radiological examinations and be subject to the same dollar limits, deductibles,
                    and coinsurance factors.

                    Law defines "low-dose mammography."

Quality Assurance   Not indicated.

Effective Date   July 1, 1981; last amendment effective July 30, 1998.

Illinois   **215 ILCS 5/356g(b)**

Scope   Reimbursement for Breast Reconstruction and Prosthesis

Policies   Law requires that all accident or health insurance policies that provide for
and Limits   mastectomy also offer coverage for prosthetic devices and reconstructive surgery
                      incident to the mastectomy, providing that the mastectomy occurred after July 1,
                      1981.

                      If, when the mastectomy is performed there is no evidence of malignancy, then
                      the offered coverage may be limited to the provision of prosthetic devices and
                      reconstructive surgery to "within 2 years after the date of the mastectomy".

                      The offered coverage is subject to deductible or coinsurance provisions applied to
                      the mastectomy and all other terms and conditions applicable to other benefits.

                      Law defines "mastectomy."

Quality Assurance   Not indicated.

Effective Date   July 1, 1981; last amendment effective June 10, 1997.

Illinois   **420 ILCS 40/5, 40/24.5, 40/25, 40/28(b)**

Scope

Accreditation of Facilities and Technologists/
Breast Cancer Screening and Education Programs

*Policies
and Limits*

Law requires all mammography procedures use a radiation machine specifically designed for and used solely for mammography. The equipment must be subjected to a quality assurance program that satisfies the quality assurance requirements of the Department.

The Department may exercise the powers, duties, and responsibilities of an accreditation body under the Mammography Quality Standards Act of 1992. The Department may implement a state program to carry out the certification program requirements provided for in the Act.

Beginning one year after the law's effective date, radiologic technologists performing mammography must satisfy training requirements established by the Department.

Unless transferred directly to the patient or physician, the provider of mammography services shall retain mammography images or films for at least 60 months. Physicians receiving films or images shall retain them for at least 60 months.

Mammography facilities must ensure that each patient is given a pamphlet that contains information on how to perform breast self-examination, on the early detection of breast cancer, and on public health facilities that can provide breast examinations and self-examination instructions. This pamphlet must be orally reviewed with each patient.

Effective Date

September 18, 1991; last amended July 19, 1995 and July 21, 1995.

Illinois　　　　　**20 ILCS 2310/55.70; 35 ILCS 5/507L, 5/509, 5/510**
　　　　　　　　　　　1999 ILL. ALS 107

Scope　　　　　　　Income Tax Checkoff for Breast and Cervical Cancer Research

Policies　　　　　　Law provides that Illinois shall include on its standard individual income tax
and Limits　　　　　form (beginning with taxable years ending December 31, 1999) a provision that
　　　　　　　　　　will allow a taxpayer to indicate that he or she wishes to contribute to the Penny
　　　　　　　　　　Severns Breast and Cervical Cancer Research Fund.

　　　　　　　　　　Law directs the Illinois Department of Public Health to award grants from the
　　　　　　　　　　Breast and Cervical Cancer Research Fund to eligible physicians, hospitals,
　　　　　　　　　　laboratories, educational institutions, and other organizations and persons for the
　　　　　　　　　　conduct of research. Research includes expenditures to develop and advance the
　　　　　　　　　　understanding, techniques, and modalities effective in the prevention, screening,
　　　　　　　　　　early detection, treatment, and cure of breast and cervical cancer and may
　　　　　　　　　　include clinical trials.

　　　　　　　　　　The Breast and Cervical Cancer Research Fund may include tax checkoff
　　　　　　　　　　receipts and gifts, grants, and awards from private foundations, nonprofit
　　　　　　　　　　organizations, and other governmental entities and persons.

　　　　　　　　　　Law directs the Department to create an advisory committee to include members
　　　　　　　　　　from the Illinois Chapter of the American Cancer Society, Y-Me, and the State
　　　　　　　　　　Board of Health.

Quality Assurance　Not indicated.

Effective Date　　　July 14, 1993; last amendment effective July 13, 1999.

Illinois   **65 ILCS 5/10-4-2.3, 105 ILCS 5/10-22.3ꜰ, 215 ILCS 5/356ᴛ, 305 ILCS 375/6.9**

Scope   Reimbursement for Inpatient Care following Mastectomy

Policies   Law requires insurers that provide surgical coverage to provide coverage for
and Limits   post-mastectomy inpatient care for a length of time determined by the attending
                 physician to be medically necessary, and based upon scientific evidence,
                 consultation with the patient, and the availability of coverage for a post-
                 discharge physician office visit or an in-home nurse to verify the patient's
                 condition within the first 48 hours after discharge.

                 This law applies to self-insuring municipalities providing health coverage to
                 employees; state employees group insurance policies of group and individual
                 accident and health insurance; and the state medical assistance program.

Quality Assurance   Not indicated.

Effective Date   June 10, 1997.

Illinois   **625 ILCS 5/3-643**

Scope   Fund for Breast Cancer Programs

Policies   Law authorizes the issuance of special registration plates designated as
and Limits   Mammogram license plates. The special plates may be issued as vanity plates or
                      personalized and shall be affixed only to passenger vehicles of the first division
                      and motor vehicles of the second division.

                      Law requires the following phrases to be on the license plates:
                      (i) "Mammograms Save Lives" and (ii) "The Susan G. Komen Foundation".

                      Law assigns the issuance and renewal fees for the Mammogram license plates.
                      Funds derived from the proceeds shall be deposited into the Mammogram Fund
                      and the Secretary of State Special License Plate Fund.

                      Law creates the Mammogram fund as a special fund in the State Treasury. All
                      money in the Mammogram Fund shall be paid as grants to the Susan G. Komen
                      Foundation for breast cancer research, education, screening, and treatment.

Quality Assurance   Not indicated.

Effective Date   January 1, 1999

Indiana   BURNS IND. CODE ANN. §§ 20-10.1-4-13

Scope   Breast Cancer Early Detection Instruction in Public Schools

Policies
and Limits   Law requires high school health education curriculum to include instruction regarding breast cancer, including the significance of early detection through monthly self breast examinations and regularly-scheduled mammographies.

Law requires the Department of Education to: (i) develop breast cancer educational materials to be made available to school corporations to assist teachers assigned to teach the material, and (ii) develop guidelines for instruction to assist teachers assigned to teach the material.

Quality Assurance   Not indicated.

Effective Date   1992

Indiana   BURNS IND. CODE ANN. §§ 27-8-14-1 to 27-8-14-6

Scope   Reimbursement for Breast Cancer Screening

Woman's Age,   35-39   Baseline
Frequency
of Mammogram   40-49   Every 2 years, but every year for a woman at risk (a woman
                                  who has a personal history of breast cancer or biopsy-proven
                                  benign breast disease; whose mother, sister, or daughter has
                                  had breast cancer; or who has not given birth by age 30).

Policies   Law requires that any policy or contract providing for third-party payment or
and Limits   prepayment of health or medical expenses include minimum mammography
                  examination coverage.

                  Law applies to individual or group accident and sickness insurance; individual or
                  group hospital or medical service contracts; individual or group health
                  maintenance organization contracts; and individual or group Medicare
                  supplemental policies (except where preempted by federal law).

                  Law does not apply to long-term care policies or contracts.

                  Mammogram benefits may be subject to any policy or contract provisions
                  applicable generally to other services under the policy or contract.

Quality Assurance   Not indicated.

Effective Date   July 2, 1989.

Indiana   BURNS IND. CODE ANN. §§ 27-13-7-15.3

Scope   Reimbursement for Breast Cancer Screening

Woman's Age,
Frequency of
Mammogram

35-39	Baseline

- 40   Each year, for a woman at risk (a woman who has a personal history of breast cancer or biopsy-proven benign breast disease; whose mother, sister, or daughter has had breast cancer; or who has not given birth by age 30).

40+   Each year

Policies
and Limits

Law provides coverage for: (i) any additional mammography views that are required for proper evaluation; and (ii) ultrasound services, if determined medically necessary by the physician treating the enrollee.

Law applies to individual or group health maintenance organization contracts. This coverage is in addition to any benefits for X-rays, laboratory testing, or wellness examinations.

Law uses the definitions for "breast cancer screening mammography" and "woman at risk" set forth in IC 27-8-14-2 and IC 27-8-14-5.

Quality Assurance   Not indicated.

Effective Date   July 1, 1999.

| **Indiana** | BURNS IND. CODE ANN. § 5-10-8-7.2 |

Scope Reimbursement for Breast Cancer Services for Public Employees

Woman's Age, 35-39   Baseline
Frequency of
Mammogram 40-49   Each year, for a woman at risk (a woman who has a personal
history of breast cancer or biopsy-proven benign breast disease;
whose mother, sister, or daughter has had breast cancer; or
who has not given birth by age 30).

50+   Each year

Policies Law requires that self-insurance programs and health maintenance organization
and Limits contracts providing health care coverage for public employees must provide
breast cancer diagnostic, outpatient treatment, and rehabilitative services.

Law requires that the reimbursement for mammography be at a level as high as
the *lower of* that established under the Medicare Economic Index or the rate
negotiated by the contracted provider. Either the state or the employee or a
combination of both shall pay the cost of coverage.

The breast cancer diagnostic services are in addition to any benefits specifically
provided for X-rays, laboratory testing, or wellness examinations. Coverage
includes a physician's interpretation of the results.

The coverage may not be subject to dollar limits, deductibles, or coinsurance
provisions less favorable than those applying to physical illness generally.

Law defines the following terms: breast cancer diagnostic service, breast cancer
outpatient treatment services, breast cancer rehabilitative services, breast cancer
screening mammography, and mammography services provider.

Quality Assurance Mammography screening must be performed by a mammography services
provider using equipment designed for and dedicated specifically to
mammography to detect unsuspected breast cancer.

The mammography services provider must be accredited by the American
College of Radiology, meet equivalent Indiana Department of Health guidelines,
or be certified by the U.S. Department of Health and Human Services for
Medicare participation.

Effective Date June 30, 1992.

Indiana   Burns Ind. Code Ann. §§ 27-8-5-26, 27-13-7-14

Scope   Reimbursement for Breast Reconstruction and Prosthesis

Policies   Law requires all accident and sickness insurance plans and health maintenance
and Limits   organizations issued after June 30, 1997 that provide coverage for mastectomy to
also include coverage for prosthetic devices and reconstructive surgery following
mastectomy.Reconstructive surgery shall include all stages of reconstruction of
the breast on which the mastectomy was performed, as well as surgery and
reconstruction of the other breast to achieve symmetry.

Coverage of prosthetic devices or reconstructive surgery shall be subject to the
deductible and coinsurance provisions that apply to the mastectomy, as well as
all other terms and conditions applicable to other benefits. If a mastectomy is
performed and covered under this section and no evidence of disease is found,
coverage may be limited to the provision of prosthetic devices and reconstructive
surgery.

Quality Assurance   Not indicated.

Effective Date   July 1, 1997.

Iowa   IOWA CODE ANN. § 514C.4

Scope   Reimbursement for Breast Cancer Screening

Woman's Age,   35-39   Baseline
Frequency
of Mammogram   40-49   Every 2 years, but more frequently upon a physician's recommendation

                            50+   Each year

Policies   Law requires that insurers offer coverage for breast cancer screening
and Limits   mammography as part of accident and sickness policies.

                            Dollar limits, deductibles, and coinsurance factors may not be less favorable
                            than those applied to physical illness generally under the accident and sickness
                            insurance policy. This coverage is in addition to any benefits for X-rays,
                            laboratory testing, or wellness examinations.

                            Coverage includes a physician's interpretation of the results.

                            Law defines "breast cancer screening mammography" and "mammography
                            services provider."

Quality Assurance   The examination must use equipment designed by the manufacturer for and
                            dedicated specifically to mammography in order to detect unsuspected breast
                            cancer. The mammography service provider must be accredited by the American
                            College of Radiology, meet equivalent State Department of Health guidelines, or
                            be certified by the U.S. Department of Health and Human Services for Medicare
                            participation.

Effective Date   July 1, 1991.

Iowa   IOWA CODE ANN. § 136C.15

Scope   Accreditation of Facilities

Policies   Law requires registration of all radiation machines used for mammography.
and Limits   Machines must be specifically authorized for use for mammography. The
                 authorization is effective for 3 years.

                 The Department shall annually inspect radiation machines.

                 Radiation equipment must meet the criteria for the American College of
                 Radiology Mammography Accreditation Program, meet the Department's
                 requirements, have an annual on-site consultation by a qualified radiation
                 physicist, be used according to Department rules on exposure and dose levels,
                 and be operated by qualified individuals.

Effective Date October 1, 1992.

Kansas   KAN. STAT. ANN. §§ 40-2229, 40-2230

Scope   Reimbursement for Breast Cancer Screening

Woman's Age,   Not stipulated.
Frequency
of Mammogram

Policies   Law requires health insurers to reimburse for mammograms only if the policy
and Limits   already covers laboratory or X-ray services. Law states that reimbursement shall
                  not be denied for mammograms when performed at the direction of a physician.

                  Law applies to individual, group, or blanket policies of accident and sickness; to
                  medical or surgical expense coverage; and to health maintenance organization
                  contracts.

                  Law does not apply to Medicare supplement policies, policies of long-term care,
                  specified accident, and accident-only coverage.

                  Deductibles, coinsurance, and other limitations apply to these benefits.

Quality Assurance   Coverage includes services performed at a mobile facility certified by the federal
                  Health Care Financing Administration and performing mammography testing by
                  American Cancer Society guidelines.

Effective Date   July 1, 1988.

Kansas KAN. STAT. ANN. § 65-2836(m)

Scope   Alternative Therapies/
                            Breast Cancer Screening and Education Programs

Policies   Law requires a physician to inform a patient suffering from any form of
and Limits   abnormality of the breast tissue for which surgery is recommended, of alternative
                            methods of treatment specified in the standardized summary distributed by the
                            licensing authority.

Quality Assurance   Not indicated.

Effective Date   Before 1993.

Kentucky   **KRS §§ 214.550 to 214.556**

Scope   Breast Cancer Screening and Education Programs/
                     Fund for Breast Cancer Screening

Policies   Law establishes the Breast Cancer Screening Fund and Breast Cancer Screening
and Limits   Program to reduce morbidity and mortality from breast cancer in women through
                     early detection and treatment, and to make screening services of high quality and
                     reasonable cost available to women of all income levels and to those whose
                     economic circumstances or geographical location limits access to breast cancer
                     screening facilities. Screening services under the program may be undertaken by
                     private contract or operated by the Kentucky Department of Health Services. The
                     program may also provide referral services.

                     The Department may adopt a schedule of income-based fees for breast cancer
                     screening. Where practical, the Department may collect any available insurance
                     proceeds or other reimbursement. The Department may accept grants or awards
                     of funds from federal or private sources.

                     The law creates a breast cancer advisory committee to develop guidelines.

                     The law creates the Kentucky Cancer Registry and the cancer patient data
                     management system.

Quality Assurance   Not indicated.

Effective Date   July 1, 1990.

Kentucky   **KRS §§ 304.17-316, 304.18-098, 304.32-1591, 304.38-1935**

Scope   Reimbursement for Breast Cancer Screening

Woman's Age,   35-39   Baseline
Frequency
of Mammogram   40-49   Every 2 years

                    50+   Each year

Policies   Law requires insurers to reimburse for low-dose mammography screening if the
and Limits   policy covers surgical services for mastectomies.

                    Law applies to individual, group, and blanket health insurance policies; health
                    maintenance organizations; and nonprofit hospital, medical-surgical, dental, and
                    health service corporations.

                    Coverage may be limited to $50 per screening.

                    Law defines "mammogram."

Quality Assurance Mammogram must be performed on equipment specifically dedicated to
                    mammography. Average radiation exposure must meet levels recommended in
                    guidelines of the American College of Radiology.

                    Law defines who may perform screening (American College of Radiology
                    certification), procedures, and equipment. Facilities performing mammograms
                    must meet American College of Radiology Mammography Accreditation
                    Program guidelines.

Effective Date   October 15, 1990.

Kentucky **KRS §§ 304.17-3163, 304.17A-134, 304.18-0983, 304.32-1593, 304.38-1934**

Scope Reimbursement for Breast Reconstruction and Prosthesis

Policies and Limits Law requires health insurers covering surgical expenses for mastectomies to also provide coverage for all stages of breast reconstruction surgery following a mastectomy that resulted from breast cancer.

Law applies to individual, group, or blanket policies and certificates; contracts issued by nonprofit hospital, medical-surgical, dental, and health service corporations; contracts issued by health maintenance organizations; and benefits provided by health benefit plans.

Law states that insurers shall not offer coverage for mastectomies that requires the procedure be performed on an outpatient basis.

Quality Assurance Not indicated.

Effective Date July 15, 1998

Kentucky   **KRS § 311.935**

Scope   Alternative Therapies/Breast Cancer Screening and Education Programs

Policies   Law directs the McDowell Cancer Network, Inc., and the James Graham Brown
and Limits   Cancer Center to jointly develop and periodically update a standardized written
summary of the advantages, disadvantages, risks, and descriptions of all
medically efficacious and viable breast cancer treatment alternatives. The
summary, to be submitted to the Kentucky Cabinet for Human Resources, must
be in layman's language, and in language understood by the patient.

Law provides that the Cabinet print and make available copies of the summary
for distribution by physicians to patients.

Law requires physicians to provide the summary to breast cancer patients.

Quality Assurance   Not indicated.

Effective Date   July 13, 1984.

Kentucky   **KRS § 304.17-3165, 304.17a-135, 304.18-0985,**
                      304.32-1595, 304.38-1936

Scope   Reimbursement for Chemotherapy and Bone Marrow Transplant for Breast
                      Cancer

Policies   Law requires health insurance plans, policies, certificates, and contracts that
and Limits   provide coverage for the treatment of breast cancer by chemotherapy on an
                      expense-incurred basis to provide coverage for such treatment by high-dose
                      chemotherapy with autologous bone marrow transplantation or stem cell
                      transplantation.

                      Law applies to individual, group, or blanket policies and certificates; contracts
                      issued by nonprofit hospital, medical-surgical, dental, and health service
                      corporations; contracts issued by health maintenance organizations; and benefits
                      provided by health benefit plans.

                      This coverage shall not be subject to any greater coinsurance or copayment than
                      that applicable to any other coverage provided by the plan.

Quality Assurance   High-dose chemotherapy with transplantation shall only be covered when
                      administered in institutions that comply with the guidelines of the American
                      Society for Blood and Marrow Transplantation or the International Society of
                      Hematotherapy and Graft Engineering, whichever has the higher standard.

Effective Date   March 28, 1996.

Louisiana   **LA. R.S. § 17:275**

Scope   Breast Cancer Early Detection Instruction in Public Schools

Policies   Law requires public junior and senior high schools to provide instruction to all
and Limits   female students in the proper procedure for breast self-examination. Such
instruction may be provided in the context of courses in the study of health,
physical education, or such other appropriate curriculum or instruction period,
as may be determined by the respective local health school boards.

Law requires the instruction to be taught by a school nurse, physician, or
competent medical instructor.

Law authorizes the local school boards to adopt rules and regulations necessary
for the implementation of the program.

Law provides that a student, whose parent or tutor submits a written statement
indicating that such instruction conflicts with the religious beliefs of the student,
shall not be required to take such instruction.

Quality Assurance   Not indicated.

Effective Date   August 1, 1980.

Louisiana   **LA. R.S. § 46:975; 2000 LA. ACT 131; 2000 LA. HB 153**

Scope   Breast Cancer Screening and Education Program

Policies   Law establishes the Breast Cancer Control Program within the Women's Health
and Limits   Program Office of Public Health to concentrate on breast cancer detection,
                      prevention, and treatment.

                      Law requires the program to provide minimum mammography examinations,
                      services, and education necessary to prevent or reduce the occurrence of breast
                      cancer and increase the statewide mammography source.

                      Law defines "minimum mammography examination" as mammographic
                      examinations performed no less frequently than the following schedule provides:

                      # One baseline mammogram for any person who is 35 through 39 years of age.

                      # One mammogram every 2 years for any person who is 40 through 49 years of
                      age, or more frequently if recommended by her physician.

                      # One mammogram each year for any person who is 50 years of age or older.

                      Law gives the Department of Health and Hospitals regulatory authority to
                      implement the program.

                      Law states that the program shall be funded through the Health Excellence Fund
                      and the Louisiana Fund (Tobacco Settlement).

Quality Assurance   Not indicated.

Effective Date   June 6, 2000.

Louisiana   LA. R.S. § 22:215.11

Scope   Reimbursement for Breast Cancer Screening

Woman's Age,   35-39   Baseline
Frequency
of Mammogram   40-49   Every 24 months, or more frequently upon physician's
                                      recommendation

                       50+   Every 12 months

Policies   Law requires insurers to include benefits payable for mammography
and Limits   examination.

                       Law applies to hospital, health, medical expense insurance policies; the state
                       employees' group benefit program (effective July 1, 1998); hospital or medical
                       service contracts; employee welfare benefit plans; health and accident insurance
                       policies; or any other insurance contract of this type. Excepted are limited benefit
                       and supplemental health insurance policies.

                       The benefits are payable under the same circumstances and conditions as benefits
                       paid under the policies for all other diagnoses, illnesses, or accidents.

                       Law defines "minimum mammography examination."

Quality Assurance   Not indicated.

Effective Date   January 1, 1992; amended by 1997 La. Act 1439, July 15, 1997.

Louisiana   **1997 LA. ALS 1341; 1997 LA. ACT 1341; 1997 LA. SB 699**

Scope   Reimbursement for Breast Reconstruction and Prosthesis

Policies   Law states that insurance policies covering mastectomy surgery must also cover
and Limits   reconstruction of the breast on which surgery has been performed and
                 reconstruction of the other breast to produce a symmetrical appearance.
                 Coverage shall be subject to those surgeries that are part of a treatment plan
                 agreed to by the patient and the attending physician. Coverage is only required if
                 the reconstructive surgery is performed under the same policy or plan that the
                 mastectomy was performed.

                 Coverage is subject to the same deductible, coinsurance, and copayment
                 provisions applicable to mastectomy surgery.

                 Law applies to hospital, health, or medical expense policies; hospital or medical
                 service contracts; employee welfare benefit plans; health and accident insurance
                 policies; group insurance plans; the state employees' group benefits program;
                 self-insurance plans; health maintenance organizations; preferred provider
                 organizations; and any policy of group, family group, blanket, or franchise
                 health and accident insurance.

                 Law does not apply to individually underwritten limited benefit and
                 supplemental health insurance policies.

Quality Assurance   Not indicated.

Effective Date   January 1, 1998.

Louisiana   LA. R.S. §§ 40:1300.151 TO 40:1300.154

Scope   Alternative Therapies/Informed Consent for Breast Cancer Treatment

Policies   Law requires the Department of Health and Hospitals, in consultation with the
and Limits   Louisiana Cancer and Lung Trust Fund Board to develop a standard, written
                      summary, using layman's terminology, of the advantages, disadvantages, risks,
                      and descriptions of the procedures regarding medically viable and efficacious
                      alternative methods of treatment for breast cancer, including surgical,
                      radiological, or chemotherapeutic treatments or combinations thereof.

                      Law requires physicians who are treating patients with any form of breast cancer
                      to inform the patient, orally and in writing, of the alternative efficacious methods
                      of treatment by discussing such alternative methods of treatment with the patient
                      and by providing the patient with the written summary.

                      Law requires the physician or surgeon to indicate on the patient's medical chart
                      the date and time that he or she has discussed alternative methods of treatment
                      with the patient and has given the patient the summary.

Quality Assurance   Law requires the Department to review and, if necessary, to revise the summary
                      every 3 years. If the department determines that new or revised information
                      should be included in the summary, the department shall revise the summary
                      prior to the 3-year review.

                      Law requires the Louisiana State Board of Medical Examiners to make printed
                      copies of the summary available to physicians and surgeons upon their request.
                      The Board is also required to establish a distribution system for the summary
                      that is linked to the renewal of a physician's license.

                      Law states that the failure of a physician or surgeon to discuss such alternative
                      methods of treatment with his patient or to provide the summary to his patient
                      shall be considered unprofessional conduct.

Effective Date   July 1, 2000

Louisiana   **LA. R.S. § 47:120.61**

Scope   Income Tax Checkoff for Breast Cancer Funds

Policies   Law directs that state income tax returns contain a checkoff allowing every
and Limits   individual, who files an individual income tax return for the current tax year and
                    who is entitled to a refund, to contribute all or any portion of the total amount of
                    the refund to the Louisiana Breast Cancer Task Force.

                    Donations shall be forwarded to the Louisiana Breast Cancer Task Force
                    annually.

                    Law requires a central record to be kept with the amount of the individual
                    donations and the name of the donors.

Quality Assurance Not indicated.

Effective Date   June 9, 1999

Maine   **24 M.R.S. §§ 2320-A, 2745-A, 2837-A, 4237-A**

Scope   Reimbursement for Breast Cancer Screening

Woman's Age,   40+   At least once a year
Frequency
of Mammogram

Policies   Law requires health insurers to provide reimbursement coverage for screening
and Limits   mammography.

                             Law applies to all individual, group, and blanket health insurance policies that
                             provide coverage for radiologic procedures. Law also applies to individual and
                             group nonprofit hospitals, medical service organizations, and health maintenance
                             organizations that meet standards established by the Department of Human
                             Services radiation protection rules.

                             Law does not apply to policies that cover only dental, accident, or specific
                             disease.

                             Law requires insurers to submit data on claims paid. The Maine Superintendent
                             of Insurance shall submit a report to the Mandated Benefits Advisory Committee.

                             Law defines "screening mammography."

Quality Assurance   Providers must meet Maine Department of Human Services' standards relating to
                             radiation protection.

Effective Date   March 1, 1991; last amended January 1, 1998.

Maine   **24 M.R.S. §§ 2332-G, 4241**
                   24-A M.R.S. § 2847-F

Scope   Reimbursement for Breast Cancer Screening

Woman's Age,   Not stipulated.
Frequency
of Mammogram

Policies   Law requires insurers to cover annual gynecological examinations that include
and Limits   clinical breast examinations.

                   Law applies to managed care plans that require enrollees to select primary care
                   physicians. Such plans may be group policies or contracts issued by health
                   maintenance organizations; insurers; or nonprofit hospital and medical service
                   organizations.

Quality Assurance The examinations may be performed by physicians, certified nurse practitioners,
                   or certified nurse midwives participating in the plan, without prior approval from
                   the primary care physician. The plan may require that patients obtain referrals
                   from their primary care physician for any follow-up care.

Effective Date   Last amended 1997.

Maine **24 M.R.S. §§ 2320-C, 2745-C, 2837-C, 4237**

Scope Reimbursement for Breast Reconstruction and Prosthesis

Policies Law states that insurance policies covering mastectomy surgery must also cover
and Limits reconstruction of the breast on which surgery has been performed and
reconstruction of the other breast to produce a symmetrical appearance. This
coverage is required if the patient elects reconstruction, and applies to
reconstruction performed in the manner chosen by the patient and the physician,
and is determined to be medically appropriate by both.

Health insurance policies may not modify the terms and conditions based on an
enrollee's request for less than the minimum coverage required under this law.
Additionally, the law directs policies to provide written notice of the coverage
required and to display the information prominently in plan literature or
correspondence.

Law applies to individual and group nonprofit and medical services plan
contracts; nonprofit health care plan contracts; individual and group health
policies; and other specified individual and group coverage.

Law does not apply to accidental injury, specified disease, Medicare supplement,
and other limited benefit policies and contracts

Quality Assurance Not indicated.

Effective Date 1995 enactment; amended January 1, 1998.

Maine

24 M.R.S. § 2905A

Scope   Alternative Therapies/Informed Consent for Breast Cancer Treatment

Policies   Law requires that physicians who are administering primary treatment for breast
and Limits   cancer must inform the patient, orally and in writing, about alternative,
efficacious methods of treating breast cancer, including surgery, radiologic
treatments, or chemotherapy, as well as the advantages, disadvantages, and risks
of each of these treatments.

Written information used may be either a standard, written summary developed
by the State Bureau of Health after consultation with the Cancer Advisory
Committee, or a brochure that is approved or distributed by the National Cancer
Institute, the American Cancer Society, the American College of Surgeons, or
any other recognized professional organization approved by the Bureau of
Health. Patients must sign a form indicating that they have received the required
oral information, and a copy of the brochure or written summary that they
receive shall be included in their medical record.

Nothing in this section shall restrict the rights of a patient under common law.

Quality Assurance   Not indicated.

Effective Date   1989.

Maine   **24 M.R.S. §§ 2320-C, 2745-C, 2837-C, 4237**

Scope   Reimbursement for Inpatient Care Following Mastectomy

Policies   Law enacts the Breast Cancer Patient Protection Act. Law requires that inpatient
and Limits   care subsequent to a mastectomy, lumpectomy, or lymph node dissection for the
                     treatment of breast cancer be provided for a period of time determined to be
                     medically appropriate by the attending physician in consultation with the patient.

                     Law does not require the provision of specified inpatient coverage if the
                     physician and patient determine that a shorter length of stay is appropriate.

                     Health insurance policies may not modify the terms and conditions based on an
                     enrollee's request for less than the minimum coverage required under this law.
                     Additionally, the law directs policies to provide written notice of the coverage
                     required and to display the information prominently in plan literature or
                     correspondence.

                     Law applies to individual and group nonprofit and medical services plan
                     contracts; nonprofit health care plan contracts; individual and group health
                     policies; and other specified individual and group coverage.

                     Law does not apply to accidental injury, specified disease, Medicare supplement,
                     and other limited benefit policies and contracts.

Quality Assurance Not indicated.

Effective Date   January 1, 1998.

Maine   **22 M.R.S. § 8711.2**

Scope   Reporting Requirements for Mammography Services

Policies   Law authorizes and directs the Maine Health Data Organization to require
and Limits   mammography providers to furnish specified data to the Organization.
                             Information that may be collected includes the locations of mammography units;
                             purchases of new mammography units; numbers of screening and diagnostic
                             mammograms performed; charges per mammogram; methods and amounts of
                             payments; and numbers of cancers detected by screening mammograms.

                             These data are to assist in evaluations of the social and financial impact and the
                             efficacy of the mandated benefit for screening mammograms.

Quality Assurance   Not indicated.

Effective Date   May 1, 1996.

Maryland   MD. HEALTH-GENERAL CODE ANN. § 20-116

Scope   Breast Cancer Screening and Education Programs/
            Reimbursement for Breast Cancer Screening

Woman's Age,   40-49   At least every 2 years
Frequency
of Clinical Breast   50+   Every year
Examination and
Mammogram

Policies and Limits   Law requires the creation, by the Department of Health and Mental Hygiene,
                          of a Breast Cancer Program to provide screening mammograms and clinical
                          breast examinations to specified low-income, underinsured and low-income,
                          uninsured women.

                          Law also requires the Program to provide diagnosis and treatment for individuals
                          who are identified as being in need or requiring specified funding.

                          Law requires the Department to administer the Program through the local health
                          departments using a grant program under which a local health department makes
                          arrangements with health care facilities to provide screening mammograms and
                          clinical breast examinations to eligible individuals.

                          Law states that for each fiscal year, an appropriation of general funds to the
                          Program shall be made.

                          Law defines "clinical breast examination" and "mammogram."

Quality Assurance   Not indicated.

Effective Date   July 1, 1998.

Maryland   MD. ANN. CODE § 19-348

Scope   Breast Cancer Screening and Education Programs

Policies   Law requires hospitals to offer mammography educational materials to each
and Limits   female patient when it is medically appropriate for the patient. The Department
                     of Health and Mental Hygiene shall select (or develop), print, and update these
                     materials, in collaboration with the Maryland Hospital Association, the Medical
                     and Chirurgical Faculty of Maryland, and appropriate advocacy groups.

Quality Assurance Not indicated.

Effective Date   October 1, 1996.

Maryland   Mᴅ. HEALTH-GENERAL Cᴏᴅᴇ Aɴɴ. § 18-303

Scope   Breast Cancer Screening Program

Policies   Law provides for a statewide public information campaign on diethylstilbestrol
and Limits   (DES) to reach individuals who have been exposed to diethylstilbestrol and each
                     offspring of those individuals, to encourage them to seek medical care for the
                     prevention or treatment of cancer that results from the exposure to
                     diethylstilbestrol.

                     Law requires an expansion of the existing cancer screening programs to detect
                     any cancer or other abnormal condition that results from exposure to
                     diethylbestrol, including breast cancer.

                     Law requires the establishment of a program to train physicians, physician's
                     assistants, and nurses in: (i) identifying individuals who have been exposed to
                     diethylstilbestrol; (ii) diagnosing and treating any cancer or other abnormal
                     condition that results from the exposure; and (iii) preventing exposure to
                     diethylstilbestrol.

                     Law states that a sliding fee schedule *may* be set for services provided. The state
                     shall reimburse a provider of screening and diagnosis in the amount that the
                     screening and diagnosis exceeds the total of the fee charged for the service and of
                     all third party payments for the service.

Quality Assurance Not indicated.

Effective Date   Last amendment effective June 1, 1995.

Maryland   MD. INSURANCE CODE ANN. § 15-814;
                 MD. INSURANCE CODE ANN. § 15-907

Scope   Reimbursement for Breast Cancer Screening

Woman's Age,   35-39   Baseline
Frequency
of Mammogram   40-49   Every 2 years, or more frequently upon physician's
                         recommendation

                 50+   Every year

Policies   Law requires insurers to provide coverage for mammograms.
and Limits
                 Law applies to nonprofit health service plans; hospital or major medical insurance
                 policies; and group or blanket health insurance policies. Medicare supplemental
                 policies are required to cover low dose mammography if allowed by amendment
                 of § 1882 (p) of the federal Social Security Act.

                 An insurer may not impose a deductible on the coverage required under this law.

                 Beginning July 30, 1993, insurers must annually report to the Insurance
                 Commissioner, for forwarding to the Interdepartmental Committee on Mandated
                 Insurance Benefits, screening mammogram information on average charges,
                 average allowed charge, average payout, total number of women covered by age
                 categories, total number of screening mammograms per year by age categories,
                 total amount paid, and total amount paid for the treatment of cancer by stage of
                 disease and age categories.

                 Law defines the following terms: mammogram, screening mammogram, and low-
                 dose mammography.

Quality Assurance An insurer has no obligation to cover screening mammograms provided by a
                 facility that is not accredited by the American College of Radiology or not
                 certified or licensed under a program established by the state.

Effective Date July 1, 1991.

Maryland   MD. INSURANCE CODE ANN. § 15-815
                 MD. HEALTH-GENERAL CODE ANN. § 19-706(d)

Scope   Reimbursement for Breast Reconstruction and Prosthesis

Policies   Law requires that insurers provide coverage for reconstructive breast surgery.
and Limits   This coverage includes all stages of reconstructive surgery performed on a
                           nondiseased breast to establish symmetry with a diseased breast when
                           reconstructive surgery is performed on the diseased breast.

                           Law applies to health maintenance organizations, and to insurers or nonprofit
                           health service plans that provide hospital, medical, or surgical benefits to any
                           group or individual on an expense-incurred basis.

                           Law defines "mastectomy" and "reconstructive breast surgery."

Effective Date   October 1, 1996, for new policies; October 1, 1997, for policies in effect before
                           October 1, 1996; last amended 1997.

Scope   Reimbursement for Breast Reconstruction and Prosthesis

Policies   Law requires that for a patient who receives less than 48 hours of inpatient
and Limits   hospitalization following a mastectomy, or who undergoes a mastectomy on an
                           outpatient basis, insurers must provide coverage for the following:
                           (i) one home visit within 24 hours after hospital discharge or outpatient health
                           care facility; and (ii) an additional home visit if prescribed by the patient's
                           attending physician.

                           Law applies to health maintenance organizations, and to insurers or nonprofit
                           health service plans that provide hospital, medical, or surgical benefits to any
                           group or individual on an expense-incurred basis.

Quality Assurance   Law defines "mastectomy."

Effective Date   October 1, 1999, for new policies; October 1, 2000, for policies in effect before
                           October 1, 1999.

Maryland   MD. HEALTH-GENERAL CODE ANN. § 20-115

Scope   Accreditation of Facilities and Technologists

Policies   Law requires that individuals performing mammography testing be qualified
and Limits   under the Maryland Health Occupation Article. In addition, testing centers must
                      be accredited under the American College of Radiology Screening
                      Mammography Accreditation Program and have a certificate of approval from
                      the federal Food and Drug Administration as specified in the Mammography
                      Quality Standards Act of 1992.

                      Law defines "mammogram" and "mammography testing."

Effective Date   July 1, 1992; last amended October 1, 1996.

Scope   Alternative Therapies/Breast Cancer Screening and Education Programs

Policies   Law requires that before treating any patient for any form of breast cancer, the
and Limits   physician shall educate the patient on alternative methods of treatment. Use of
                     the Maryland Department of Health and Mental Hygiene's standardized written
                     summary satisfies this requirement.

                     Law directs that the Department provide a standardized written summary, in
                     layman's language, that lists all effective methods of treatment for breast cancer
                     that may be medically practicable and describes the advantages, disadvantages,
                     risks, and procedures associated with each method of treatment listed.

                     Law does not apply for treatment occurring within 5 days of diagnosis or
                     treatment necessary to save the patient's life.

Quality Assurance Not indicated.

Effective Date   1986 enactment; last amended 1990.

Massachusetts   **1997 MASS. ALS 43; 1997 MASS. H.B. 4700**

Scope   Breast Cancer Screening and Education Programs/Breast Cancer Research
                         Programs

Policies   Law directs the Massachusetts Department of Public Health to conduct a   study
and Limits   and file a report on a 5-year program for breast cancer prevention, research and
                         detection services. The report is to incorporate and evaluate the results of the
                         scientific research grant program investigating potential   environmental
                         factors that contribute to breast cancer in areas of "unique opportunity."

                         Law also provides for an early breast cancer detection program, mammographies
                         for the uninsured, breast cancer research, and a breast cancer detection public
                         awareness program.

Quality Assurance   Not indicated.

Effective Date   Enacted upon passage, July 10, 1997.

Massachusetts   MASS. GEN. LAWS ANN. CH. 111 § 4K

Scope   Breast Cancer Screening Program

Policies   Law requires the establishment, promotion, and maintenance of a statewide
and Limits   public information program regarding diethylstilbestrol (DES).

Law requires the program to designate and enter into contracts with providers of
health care for the purpose of establishing regional screening programs for
women who were exposed to DES during pregnancy and their offspring who
were exposed prenatally.

Law requires consideration of providers' compliance with state and federally
mandated standards, the location in relation to the geographic distribution of
persons exposed to DES, and the capacity of the provider to properly screen for
breast cancer and any other malignancy and abnormal conditions resulting from
DES exposure.

Law requires the establishment of a program to train physicians, physician's
assistants, and nurses in the detection, diagnosis, treatment, and prevention of
diseases in women who were exposed to DES during pregnancy and their
offspring who were exposed prenatally.

Quality Assurance   Not indicated.

Effective Date   Last amendment effective June 6, 1997.

Massachusetts   M ASS. G EN. L AWS A NN. Ch. 175 §§ 47G, 110; Ch. 176A § 8J; Ch. 176B § 4I; Ch. 176G § 4

Scope   Reimbursement for Breast Cancer Screening

Woman's Age,   35-40   Baseline
Frequency
of Mammogram   40+   Each year

Policies   Law applies to blanket or general accident or sickness and employer's health and
and Limits   welfare fund policies; individual group hospital service plans; individual or group medical service agreements; and health maintenance organizations.

Law does not apply to Medicare supplemental insurance polices.

Quality Assurance   Not indicated.

Effective Date   November 27, 1987.

Massachusetts   **MASS. GEN. LAWS ANN. Ch. 111 § 5Q**

Scope   Accreditation of Facilities

Policies   Law directs the Massachusetts Department of Public Health to promulgate rules
and Limits   and regulations for the licensing of mammography facilities.

                       The rules shall be as stringent as the most current standards of the American
                       College of Radiology and require that a physician be designated by the facility as
                       responsible for overall quality assurance.

                       Rules and regulations shall also include optimum exposure ranges, equipment
                       standards and requirements, mandated quality assurance programs, phantom
                       image quality requirements, operator training and experience requirements,
                       annual evaluation and calibration of the mammography unit by a qualified
                       radiation physicist, registration of mammography facility and specific inspection
                       procedures by Department inspectors, and reporting and record keeping
                       requirements. In lieu of the above, the Department may accept certification by
                       the American College of Radiology or other recognized organization.

                       Mammograms must be read and interpreted by a physician.

                       The radiologic technologist is responsible for ensuring that the radiographs meet
                       the technical and diagnostic requirements of the physician reading the
                       mammogram.

                       The Department shall require the use of radiographic systems specifically
                       designed for and exclusively used for mammography.

                       The Department shall inspect mammography facilities annually.

                       The Department may suspend or revoke a license of a facility violating this law.

Effective Date   October 18, 1992.

| **Massachusetts** | **MASS. GEN. LAWS ANN. CH. 175 § 47M; 176A § 8O; CH. 176B § 4O; CH. 176G § 4F; CH. 32A § 17D; CH. 175 § 47R** |

Scope   Reimbursement for Bone Marrow Transplant for Breast Cancer

Policies and Limits

Law requires insurers to provide coverage for bone marrow transplant or transplants for persons who have been diagnosed with breast cancer that has progressed to metastatic disease.

Law applies to accident and health insurance policies; non-profit hospital service corporations; medical service corporations; health maintenance contracts; and policies covering active or retired employees of the Commonwealth.

Patients must meet criteria established by the Massachusetts Department of Public Health consistent with medical research protocols reviewed and approved the National Cancer Institute.

Quality Assurance   Not indicated.

Effective Date   April 13, 1994; amended December 27, 1996.

Massachusetts   MASS. GEN. LAWS ANN. Ch. 71 § 1

Scope   Breast Cancer Early Detection Instruction in Public Schools

Policies   Law directs that public school health education programs include instruction on
and Limits   the detection and prevention of breast cancer.

Quality Assurance   Not indicated.

Effective Date   1977 enactment.

Michigan   **M.C.L. §§ 333.9501, 333.9503**

Scope   Breast Cancer Screening and Education Programs/Accreditation of Facilities

Policies   Law establishes the Breast Cancer Mortality Reduction Program, which
and Limits   includes:

                  # professional skills education programs for health professionals to develop
                  state-of-the-art skills in screening, diagnosis, referral, treatment, and
                  rehabilitation.

                  # public education programs on the benefits of regular screening; the procedures
                  that can make the best use of the medical care systems for screening, diagnosis,
                  referral, treatment, and rehabilitation; and treatment options for cancer.

                  # applied research and community demonstration grant programs for local
                  communities to demonstrate and evaluate the best methods to reduce cancer
                  morbidity and mortality and to provide access to breast cancer screening,
                  diagnosis, treatment, and rehabilitation services for populations with higher than
                  expected rates of breast cancer morbidity or mortality.

Quality Assurance The Michigan Department of Health will promulgate rules for licenses or
                  registration for radioactive materials, and for registration of machines to perform
                  mammographies. The law provides quality assurance (American College of
                  Radiology Mammography Accreditation Program) criteria for machines and
                  facilities.

Effective Date Last amended 1989.

Michigan   **M.C.L. §§ 333.21054a, 500.3406d, 500.3616, 550.1416**

Scope	Reimbursement for Breast Cancer Screening

Woman's Age,	35-39	Baseline
Frequency		
of Mammogram	40+	Each year

Policies and Limits

Law requires that health maintenance organizations; hospital, medical, or surgical expense-incurred policies; and group and non-group certificates of health care corporations include coverage for breast cancer diagnostic services, breast cancer outpatient treatment services, and breast cancer rehabilitative services. Group and non-group certificates of health care corporations must cover breast cancer screening mammography.

Dollar limits, deductibles, and coinsurance provisions may not be less favorable than those for physical illness generally.

Law defines the following terms: breast cancer diagnostic services, breast cancer rehabilitative services, breast cancer screening mammography, and breast cancer outpatient treatment services.

Quality Assurance

Breast cancer screening mammography must use equipment designed and dedicated specifically for mammography in order to detect unsuspected breast cancer.

Effective Date

November 1, 1989; no subsequent amendment.

Michigan M.C.L. §§ 500.3613, 500.3406A, 550.1415

Scope Reimbursement for Breast Reconstruction and Prosthesis

Policies and Limits Law requires that hospital, medical, or surgical expense-incurred policies and group and non-group certificates of health care corporations provide benefits for prosthetic devices to maintain or replace the body part of an individual who has undergone a mastectomy.

Reasonable charges for medical care and attendance for an individual who receives reconstructive surgery following a mastectomy or who is fitted with a prosthetic device are a covered benefit after the attending physician certifies the medical necessity or desirability of a proposed course of rehabilitative treatment.

Quality Assurance Not indicated.

Effective Date March 30, 1983; no subsequent amendment.

Michigan   M.C.L. §§ 333.17013, 333.17513

Scope   Alternative Therapies/Breast Cancer Screening and Education Programs

Policies   Law directs that a physician administering primary treatment for breast cancer to
and Limits   a patient diagnosed as having breast cancer shall inform the patient, orally and in
    writing, about alternative methods of treatment. The physician also shall inform
    the patient of the advantages, disadvantages, risks, and procedures of each
    method of treatment. Use of the Michigan Department of Public Health's
    standardized written summary or brochure satisfies this requirement.

    The standardized written summary or brochure shall:

    # be developed by the Department in cooperation with the Chronic Disease
    Advisory Committee;

    # be drafted in nontechnical terms that the patient can understand;

    # inform the patients about alternative methods of treatment;

    # inform the patients about the advantages, disadvantages, and risks for each
    method of treatment and about the procedures involved in each method of
    treatment; and

    # be available to physicians through the Michigan Board of Medicine and the
    Michigan Board of Osteopathic Medicine and Surgery.

    The patient's medical record shall include the standardized written summary or a
    signed form indicating that the patient has received the brochure. A patient who
    signs the form shall be barred from subsequently bringing a civil action against
    the physician based on failure to obtain informed consent, but only in regard to
    information on alternative forms of treatment and associated advantages,
    disadvantages, and risks.

Quality Assurance   Not indicated.

Effective Date   July 8, 1986; last amendment effective May 15, 1989.

Minnesota   MINN. STAT. ANN. §§ 62A.30, 62A.315, 62A.316

Scope   Reimbursement for Breast Cancer Screening

Woman's Age,   Not stipulated.
Frequency
of Mammogram

Policies   Law requires insurers to include coverage for routine mammogram screening
and Limits   procedures.

Law applies to all policies of accident and health insurance; health maintenance
contracts; health benefit certificates of fraternal benefit societies; and subscriber
contracts of nonprofit health service plans. Under Section 62A.315, extended
basic Medicare supplement plans must cover 100 percent of the cost of routine
screening procedures for cancer, including mammograms.

Law does not apply to policies designed primarily to provide coverage payable
on a per diem, fixed indemnity, or non-expense-incurred basis, or policies that
provide only accident coverage.

Quality Assurance   Not indicated.

Effective Date   August 1, 1988; last amended 1998.

Minnesota   MINN. STAT. ANN. § 144.651(9)

Scope   Alternative Therapies

Policies   Law requires every physician provide each breast cancer patient (or Minnesota
and Limits   state resident) suffering from any form of breast cancer with fully complete and
current information about their diagnosis, treatment, alternatives, risks, and
prognosis.

Law requires such information be provided in terms and language which the
patients or residents can reasonably be expected to understand.

Such information must include any likely medical or major psychological results
of the treatment and its alternatives.

Law requires such information concerning all alternative effective methods of
treatment about which the treating physician is knowledgeable (including, but not
limited to: surgical, radiologic, chemotherapeutic treatments or combinations of
treatments, along with the risks associated with each method of treatment) be
given to the patient or resident prior to, or at the *time of admission*, and *during
her stay*.

When medically advisable, such information must be given to the patient's (or
resident's) guardian or other such person designated by the patient as her
representative.

Law mandates that the delivery of all such required information be documented,
by the attending physician, in the patient's or resident's medical record.

Quality Assurance   Not indicated.

Effective Date   1982 enactment; last amended 1999.

Minnesota　　　MINN. STAT. ANN. §§ 62A.307, 62A.309

Scope　　　Reimbursement for Chemotherapy and Bone Marrow Transplant for Breast Cancer

Policies
and Limits　　Law requires all health plans (as defined in Section 62A.011) to cover the treatment of breast cancer by high-dose chemotherapy with autologous bone marrow transplantation, and to cover expenses arising from this treatment.

This coverage shall not be subject to any greater coinsurance, copayment, or deductible than that applicable to any other coverage provided by the plan.

Quality Assurance　　Not indicated.

Effective Date　　May 19, 1995; last amended 1997.

Mississippi   MISS. CODE ANN. § 83-9-108

Scope   Reimbursement for Breast Cancer Screening

Woman's Age,   35+   Every year
Frequency
of Mammogram

Policies and Limits Law requires group or individual policies, and contracts or certificates of heath insurance issued or renewed for persons who are residents of the state, to cover screening for the presence of occult breast cancer within the provisions of the policies, contracts, or certificates. Coverage shall be offered on an optional basis, and each primary insured person must accept or reject such coverage in writing and accept responsibility for premium payment.

                       Law states that benefits under this provision shall be at least as favorable as those for other radiological examinations and subject to the same dollar limits, deductibles, and coinsurance factors.

                       Law does not apply to accident-only, specified disease (except cancer), hospital indemnity, Medicare supplement, long-term care, or limited benefit health insurance policies.

                       Law defines "low-dose mammography."

Quality Assurance   Not indicated.

Effective Date   January 1, 1999.

Missouri   **R.S.Mo., § 376.782**

Scope   Reimbursement for Breast Cancer Screening

Woman's Age,   35-39   Baseline
Frequency
of Mammogram   40-49   Every 2 years, or more frequently upon physician's
                                  recommendation

                   50+   Every year

                   Any age   Upon the recommendation of a physician, when the patient, her
                                  mother, or her sister has a prior history of breast cancer

Policies   Law requires that insurers provide coverage for low-dose mammography
and Limits   screening.

                    Law applies to individual and group health insurance policies providing coverage
                    on an expense-incurred basis; individual and group service or indemnity type
                    contracts issued by nonprofit corporations; health maintenance organization
                    individual and group service contracts; self-insured group arrangements (to the
                    extent not preempted by federal law); and managed health care delivery entities.

                    Mammography coverage and benefits shall be at least as favorable and subject to
                    the same dollar limits, deductibles, and copayments as other radiological
                    examinations.

                    Law defines "low-dose mammography."

Quality Assurance The examination must use equipment specifically designed and dedicated for
                     mammography.

Effective Date   August 28, 1990; last amended in 1995.

Missouri   **R.S.Mo., § 376.1209**

Scope   Reimbursement for Breast Reconstruction and Prosthesis

Policies   Law requires insurers to cover prosthetic devices or reconstructive surgery if
and Limits   they cover mastectomy. Coverage provided shall include devices or surgery
                   incident to the mastectomy that are recommended by the patient's oncologist or
                   primary care physician.

                   Coverage for these services shall be subject to the same deductible and
                   coinsurance conditions applied to the mastectomy and other benefits.

                   Law applies to insurers providing coverage on an expense-incurred basis,
                   contracts issued by non-profit corporations, health maintenance organizations,
                   self-insured group arrangements (to the extent allowed by federal law), and all
                   managed health care entities.

                   Law does not apply to life care contracts, accident only, specified disease, fixed
                   daily hospital benefits, Medicare supplemental, and other limited benefit policies.

                   Law defines "mastectomy."

Quality Assurance   Not indicated.

Effective Date   January 1, 1998; no subsequent amendment.

Missouri   **R.S.Mo., §§ 192.760 to 192.766**

Scope   Accreditation of Facilities

Policies   Law requires registration with the Missouri Department of Health of all radiation
and Limits   machines used for mammography. The authorization is effective for 3 years.

Law mandates annual inspections by the Department.

The radiation equipment must meet the criteria of the American College of
Radiology Mammography Accreditation Program and the Department of Health's
requirements, be specifically designed for mammography, be used exclusively for
mammography, be used in a facility that has an annual on-site consultation by a
radiation physicist, be used according to Department rules on exposure and dose
levels, and be operated by qualified individuals.

Law directs the Department of Health to issue rules on licenses or registration for
radioactive materials and other sources of ionizing radiation used to perform
mammography facilities. The rules shall provide for suspension or revocation of
licenses.

The Department may issue rules establishing requirements for record keeping,
permissible levels of exposure, notification and reports of accidents, protective
measures, technical qualifications of personnel, handling, transportation,
interpretation, storage, waste disposal, posting and labeling of hazardous sources
and areas, and surveys and monitoring.

The Department shall issue rules and regulations for a patient notification/recall
system when deficiencies are found in mammography and minimum training and
performance standards for an individual using a radiation machine for
mammography.

The rules do not limit the intentional exposure of patients to radiation for the
purpose of lawful therapy or research.

The rules may provide for recognition of other state or federal licenses.

The law provides for applications, schedule of fees, and inspections. The
Director of the Department shall deposit fees in the Mammography Fund.

Effective Date   Sixty days after August 28, 1992.

Missouri   **R.S.Mo., § 376.1200**

Scope   Reimbursement for Chemotherapy and Bone Marrow Transplant for Breast Cancer

Policies and Limits   Law requires insurers to offer coverage for the treatment of breast cancer by dose-intensive chemotherapy/autologous bone marrow transplants or stem cell transplants. The offer and acceptance must be in writing.

Law applies to entities offering individual or group health insurance policies providing coverage on an expense-incurred basis; individual and group service or indemnity contracts issued by a health services corporation; individual and group service contracts issued by a health maintenance organization; self-insured group arrangements to the extent not preempted by federal law; and managed health care delivery entities. The law does not apply to short-term travel; accident-only limited, or specified disease policies; or to short-term nonrenewable policies of not more than 7 months duration.

The coverage shall not be subject to any greater deductible or copayment than that applicable to any other coverage provided by the plan. The plan may, however, impose a lifetime benefit maximum of not less than $100,000 for dose-intensive chemotherapy/autologous bone marrow transplants.

The coverage may be administered through a managed care program of exclusive and/or preferred contractual arrangements with one or more providers. Such arrangements may hold the patient harmless for the costs of treatment in the event of a dispute between the managed care program and the provider.

Quality Assurance   Insurers are required to cover treatments only if they are performed in accordance with nationally accepted peer review protocols used by breast cancer treatment centers experienced in dose-intensive chemotherapy/autologous bone marrow transplants or stem cell transplants.

Effective Date   January 1, 1996; no subsequent amendment.

Montana   MONT. CODE ANNO., §§ 33-22-132, 53-6-101(2)(c)

Scope   Reimbursement for Breast Cancer Screening

Woman's Age,   35-39   Baseline
Frequency
of Mammogram   40-49   Every 2 years, or more frequently upon physician's
                                    recommendation

                     50+   Each year

Policies   Law requires that group or individual medical expense, cancer, and blanket
and Limits   disability policies, certificates of insurance, and membership contracts provide
                     minimum mammography examination coverage. The Montana Medicaid
                     Program includes mammography services as defined above.

                     Law does not apply to disability income, hospital indemnity, Medicare
                     supplement, accident-only, vision, dental, or specified disease policies.

                     The insurer must pay the *lesser of* $70 or the actual charge for each examination.

Quality Assurance Not indicated.

Effective Date   September 19, 1991; last amended 1997.

Montana   MONT. CODE ANNO. § 33-22-135

Scope   Reimbursement for Breast Reconstruction and Prosthesis/
                 Reimbursement for Chemotherapy

Policies   Law requires insurers to provide coverage for reconstructive surgery following
and Limits   mastectomy to include reconstructive surgery of the diseased breast, and all
                 stages of one reconstructive surgery on the non-diseased breast to establish
                 symmetry.

                 Reconstructive breast surgery coverage shall also include the costs of prostheses
                 as well as coverage for outpatient chemotherapy following surgical procedures if
                 the contract includes coverage for outpatient X-ray or radiation therapy.

                 Law applies to disability policies.

                 Law defines "mastectomy" and "reconstructive breast surgery."

Quality Assurance   Not indicated.

Effective Date   January 1, 1998; no subsequent amendment.

Montana   MONT. CODE ANNO., § 37-3-33

Scope   Alternative Therapies/Informed Consent for Breast Cancer Treatment

Policies   Law requires physicians and surgeons to secure written informed consent
and Limits   agreements from patients certifying that the patient has been informed about the
                 full range of efficacious, viable medical treatment alternatives to the removal of
                 breast tissue, including radiological or chemotherapeutic treatments or
                 combinations of these treatments; the advantages, disadvantages, risks, and
                 descriptions of the alternative procedures; and aspects of recovery including the
                 options available for reconstructive surgery.

                 Failure to provide this information to patients to the best of their available
                 knowledge constitutes unprofessional conduct on the part of the physician or
                 surgeon.

Quality Assurance   Not indicated.

Effective Date   January 1, 1998.

Montana   MONT. CODE ANNO., § 33-22-134

Scope   Reimbursement for Inpatient Care Following Mastectomy

Policies
and Limits   Law requires insurers to provide coverage for hospital inpatient care for a period of time determined necessary by the attending physician (and in the case of a health maintenance organization, also the primary care physician), in consultation with the patient, to be medically necessary following a mastectomy, lumpectomy, or lymph node dissection.

Law applies to disability policies, the state employee group insurance program, the university system employee group insurance program, employee group insurance programs in the state, and any self-funded multiple employer welfare arrangements that are not regulated by ERISA.

Quality Assurance   Not indicated.

Effective Date   January 1, 1998.

Nebraska　　　　**R.R.S. NEB. § 71-7617**

Scope　　　　　Breast Cancer Screening Program

Policies　　　　Law requires the Department of Health and Human Services to contract with the
and Limits　　　health clinics of Nebraska's federally recognized Native American tribes, Indian
　　　　　　　　health organizations, or other public health organizations that have a substantial
　　　　　　　　Native American clientele to provide breast cancer screening and early detection
　　　　　　　　services targeted to Native American populations.

Quality Assurance　Not indicated.

Effective Date　April 14, 1998.

| Nebraska | **1999 NEB. ALS 480, 1999 NEB. LAWS 480, 1999 NEB. LB 480** |

Scope Breast Cancer Screening and Education Programs/Fund for Breast Cancer Screening and Education Programs

Policies and Limits Law creates the Women's Health Initiative of Nebraska within the Department of Health and Human Services. The Women's Health Initiative of Nebraska shall strive to improve the health of women in Nebraska by fostering the development of a comprehensive system of coordinated services, policy development, advocacy, and education.

Law requires the Initiative to:

serve as a clearinghouse for information regarding women's health issues, including breast cancer.

perform strategic planning to develop department-wide plans for implementation of goals and objectives for women's health.

conduct department-wide policy analysis on specific issues related to women's health.

coordinate pilot projects and planning projects funded by the state that are related to women's health.

communicate and disseminate information to providers of health, social, educational, and support services to women.

provide technical assistance to communities, other public entities, and private entities for initiatives in women's health.

encourage innovative responses by public and private entities that are attempting to address women's health issues.

Law creates the Women's Health Initiative Advisory Council and the Women's Health Initiative Fund. The fund shall consist of money received as gifts or grants or collected as fees or charges from any federal, state, public, or private source. Money in the fund shall be used to reimburse the expenses of the Women's Health Initiative of Nebraska and expenses of members of the Women's Health Initiative Advisory Council.

Quality Assurance Not indicated.

Effective Date April 11, 2000

Nebraska   **R.R.S. Neb. §§ 44-785, 71-7001, 71-7002, 71-7003, 71-7012**

Scope

Breast Cancer Screening and Education Programs/
Reimbursement for Breast Cancer Screening

Woman's Age,
Frequency
of Mammogram

State Program:

31-49	Each year for women with a personal or family (mother or sister) history of pre-menopausal breast cancer
35-39	Baseline
40-49	Every 2 years
50-64	Each year

Insurance Mandate:

35-39	Baseline
40-49	Every 2 years, or more frequently based on a physician's recommendation
50+	Each year

Policies
and Limits

Law directs the Nebraska Department of Health to create a statewide mammography screening program, which shall reimburse mammography suppliers who provide screening mammography to eligible women. As funds permit, the program shall also provide reimbursement for definitive diagnostic procedures for women receiving abnormal screening results under the program.

Law provides that the Breast and Cervical Cancer Advisory Committee advise the Department on income guidelines for eligible women and reimbursement rates. The program will not pay for screening mammography for women who have public or private insurance covering the procedure, whose income exceeds the Department guidelines, or who are eligible for screening under any federal or state health benefit program.

Law permits the Department to receive federal and other public and private funds for the Breast and Cervical Cancer Cash Fund.

Law requires insurers to cover screening mammography, on no less favorable terms than other radiological examinations (deductibles and copayments are allowed). This mandate applies to individual or group sickness and accident policies or contracts; hospital, medical, or surgical expense-incurred policies, except specified-disease or other limited-benefit coverages; and self-funded employee benefit plans to the extent not preempted by federal law.

Quality Assurance   Mammography suppliers must meet the standards of the federal Mammography Quality Standards Act of 1992.

Effective Date   September 9, 1995. (Establishment of Breast Cancer Advisory Committee under Section 71-7012, enacted 1991; last amended 1996, effective April 4, 1996, operative January 1, 1997.)

Nebraska **R.R.S. Neb. § 71-7614**

Scope   Fund for Breast Cancer Education and Screening Programs

Policies   Law requires the Excellence in Health Care Trust Fund to be used to award
and Limits   grants for public health services which focus on education and preventive
                                 measures for breast cancer, including services for reservation or service areas of
                                 federally recognized Native American tribes in Nebraska and organizations that
                                 focus on the health of minority groups.

                                 Law creates the Excellence in Health Care Council. The Council, with the
                                 approval of the Director of Finance and Support, shall award grants to improve
                                 access to or delivery of health care services to medically underserved individuals
                                 or in medically underserved areas.

                                 Law requires recipients of such grants to provide, upon request, such data
                                 relating to the funded projects, as is deemed necessary.

Quality Assurance   Not indicated.

Effective Date   January 15, 1999; last amendment effective April 29, 1999.

Nevada   NEV. REV. STAT. §§ 689A.0405, 689B.0374, 695C.1735, 695B.1912

Scope   Reimbursement for Breast Cancer Screening

Woman's Age,   35-39   Baseline
Frequency
of Mammogram   40+   Each year

Policies   Law requires health insurers to provide coverage for mammograms.
and Limits

                 Law applies to health insurance policies; group health insurance polices; hospital or medical service corporation policies; and health maintenance plans.

                 Insurance policies and health maintenance organizations may not require insured individuals to obtain prior authorization for any of the services provided under this law.

Quality Assurance   Not indicated.

Effective Date   Enacted 1989; last amendment effective October 1, 1997.

Nevada
Nev. Rev. Stat. §§ 608.157, 616.503, 617.395, 689A.041, 689B.0375, 695B.191, 695C.171

Scope
Reimbursement for Breast Reconstruction and Prosthesis

Policies and Limits
Law requires health insurers that provide coverage for mastectomies also to provide commensurate coverage for at least two prosthetic devices and for reconstructive surgery incident to the mastectomy.

Law applies to employee health plans; workers' compensation; health insurance policies; group health insurance polices; hospital or medical service corporation policies; and health maintenance plans.

If the reconstructive surgery is begun within 3 years of the mastectomy, the amount of benefits for that surgery must equal the amount provided at the time of the mastectomy. For surgery begun more than 3 years after the mastectomy, the benefits are subject to all the terms, conditions, and exclusions in the policy at the time of the reconstructive surgery.

Law defines "reconstructive surgery."

Quality Assurance
Not indicated.

Effective Date
Enacted 1983; last amended 1989.

Nevada　　　　　NEV. REV. STAT. §§ 457.182 to 457.187

Scope　　　　Accreditation of Facilities and Technologists

Policies　　　*Radiation Machines:*
and Limits　　Law requires that a radiation machine used for mammography have a certificate of authorization from the Health Division and be accredited by the American College of Radiology or meet standards established by the Health Division. The certificate expires in one year. To obtain a certificate of authorization for a radiation machine, a person must:

submit an application to the Health Division.

provide any additional information required by the Health Division.

pay a fee.

Operators:
Law requires that a person operating a radiation machine for mammography have a valid certificate of authorization to operate the radiation machine issued by the Health Division or is licensed pursuant to statute. The certificate of authorization expires in 3 years. To obtain a certificate of authorization, a person must:

submit an application to the Health Division.

be certified by the American Registry of Radiologic Technologists or meet standards set by the Health Division.

pass any examination required by the Health Division.

pay a fee.

Effective Date　　Enacted 1991; last amended 1997.

New Hampshire	N.H. RSA §§ 417-D:1 to 417-D:4

Scope　　　Reimbursement for Breast Cancer Screening

Woman's Age, Frequency of Mammogram

35-39	Baseline
40-49	Every 1-2 years
50+	Each year

Policies and Limits

Law requires that policies of accident or health insurance providing benefits for hospital expense, medical-surgical expense, or major medical expense shall provide coverage for screening by low-dose mammography.

Benefits shall be at least as favorable as for other radiological examinations and subject to the same dollar limits, deductibles, and coinsurance factors.

Law defines "low-dose mammography."

Quality Assurance

Equipment must be dedicated specifically for mammography with a radiation exposure diagnostically valuable and in keeping with the recommended "Average Patient Exposure Guides" published by the Conference of Radiation Control Program Directors, Inc.

Effective Date

January 1, 1989; last amendment effect January 1, 1998.

New Hampshire   **N.H. RSA §§ 415:18-c, 420-A:13, 420-B:8e**

Scope   Reimbursement for Bone Marrow Transplant for Breast Cancer

Policies and Limits   Law requires any policy of group or blanket accident or health insurance provide coverage for expenses arising from the treatment of breast cancer by autologous bone marrow transplants.

Law applies to every health service corporation and every other similar corporation licensed under the laws of *another* state.

Law applies to covered individuals who are residents of the state of New Hampshire or whose principal place of business is in the state of New Hampshire.

Treatment by autologous bone marrow transplant procedure must be in accordance with protocols reviewed and approved by the National Cancer Institute.

Quality Assurance   Not indicated.

Effective Date   January 1, 1993; amended 1997.

New Jersey   N.J. STAT. §§ 26:2-168, 45:9-22.3a, 45:9-22.3b

Scope   Breast Cancer Screening and Education Programs

Policies and Limits   Law directs that the New Jersey Department of Health, in consultation with the New Jersey Division of the American Cancer Society, the Radiological Society of New Jersey, and the New Jersey Chapter of the American College of Obstetricians and Gynecologists, prepare an information booklet in English and Spanish on breast cancer prevention, detection, and treatment. The booklet must describe, in a manner easily understandable by the patient; recognized dietary and lifestyle implications for breast cancer prevention; advantages and methods of early detection; and the risks and procedures involved with alternative treatment methods.

The Department shall make the booklets available to all licensed health care facilities engaged in breast cancer diagnosis and treatment, facilities providing mammography services, physicians engaged in breast cancer diagnosis and treatment, and social service agencies that primarily serve women.

Attending physicians shall give a copy of the booklet to all patients who are referred for a routine mammogram or who are under the physician's care for treatment of breast cancer.

Quality Assurance   Not indicated.

Effective Date   Enacted 1993.

New Jersey   N.J. STAT. § 26:2-113

Scope   Breast Cancer Screening and Education Programs

Policies   Law provides for a statewide public information campaign on diethylstilbestrol
and Limits   (DES) to reach individuals who have been exposed to diethylstilbestrol and each
                     offspring of those individuals, to encourage them to seek medical care for the
                     prevention or treatment of cancer that results from the DES exposure.

                     Law requires an expansion of the existing cancer screening programs to detect
                     any cancer or other abnormal condition that results from exposure to DES,
                     including breast cancer.

                     Law requires the establishment of a program to train physicians, physician's
                     assistants, and nurses in: (i) identifying individuals who have been exposed to
                     DES; and (ii) diagnosing and treating any cancer or other abnormal condition
                     that results from the exposure.

Quality Assurance   Not indicated.

Effective Date   September 23, 1981.

New Jersey　　　**N.J. Stat. § 17B:26-2.1e, 17B:27-46.1f**

Scope　　　　Reimbursement for Breast Cancer Screening

Woman's Age,　　35-39　　　Baseline
Frequency
of Mammogram　40+　　　　Each year

Policies　　　Law requires insurers to provide coverage for mammography examination
and Limits　　benefits according to the age and frequency schedule specified above.

　　　　　　Law applies to individual or group health insurance policies that provide hospital
　　　　　　or medical expense benefits.

　　　　　　The required benefits must be provided to the same extent as for any other
　　　　　　sickness under the respective policy.

Quality Assurance　Not specified.

Effective Date　Enacted 1991; last amended 1999.

New Jersey

N.J. STAT. §§ 17:48-6b, 17-48a-7b, 17:48E-35, 17B:26-2.1a, 17B:27-46.1a, 26:2j-4.14

Scope

Reimbursement for Breast Reconstruction and Prosthesis/ Reimbursement for Chemotherapy

Policies and Limits

Law requires that health insurers provide benefits for reconstructive breast surgery including the cost of prostheses. Benefits include coverage for reconstructive surgery as well as surgery to restore symmetry between the breasts. Contracts providing outpatient X-ray or radiation therapy must also provide benefits for outpatient chemotherapy following surgical procedures for breast cancer.

Law applies to hospital service corporations, health maintenance organizations, medical service corporations, and group and blanket insurance policies.

Law applies to all contracts in which the insurer has reserved the right to change the premium.

Benefits shall be provided to the same extent as for any other sickness under the contract.

Quality Assurance

Not indicated.

Effective Date

Enacted 1983; last amended 1997.

New Jersey   N.J. STAT. ANN. §§ 52:9U-6.1, 54A:9-25.7, 54A:9-25.8

Scope   Income Tax Checkoff for Breast Cancer Research

Policies   Law directs that, beginning in 1996, state income tax returns contain a checkoff
and Limits   allowing taxpayers to contribute $5, $10, or other amounts to the New Jersey
     Breast Cancer Research Fund. The taxpayer can enclose the contribution or
     direct that it be deducted from his or her tax refund.

     Net contributions shall annually be appropriated to the New Jersey State
     Commission on Cancer Research. The Commission shall solicit, receive,
     evaluate, and approve applications for grants from the New Jersey Breast Cancer
     Research Fund. Qualified applicants include academic medical institutions, state
     or local government agencies, public or private organizations within New Jersey,
     and any other institution approved by the Commission. Grants must be used for
     scientific research projects that focus on the causes, prevention, screening,
     treatment, or cure of breast cancer.

Quality Assurance   Not indicated.

Effective Date   Enacted 1995; last amended 1998.

New Jersey   N.J. STAT. §§ 17:48-6q, 17:48A-7o, 17:48E-35.14, 17B:26-2.1m, 17B:27-46.1P, 17B:27A-7.2, 17B:27A-19.4, 26:2J-4.15, 34:13A-30, 52:14-17.29b

Scope   Reimbursement for Inpatient Stay Following a Mastectomy

Policies and Limits   Law requires insurers to provide coverage for a minimum of 72 hours of inpatient hospital care following a modified radical mastectomy and a minimum of 48 hours of inpatient care following a simple mastectomy. Contracts shall not require health care providers to obtain prior authorization for prescribing the lengths of stay required by this law as appropriate.

Law requires benefits for inpatient stay following a mastectomy to be provided to the same extent that coverage for other sicknesses is provided under the same contract.

Law is not meant to construe that patients are required to receive inpatient care for 72 or 48 hours if the patient determines that length of time is not necessary upon consultation with their physician. Law does not relieve patients and physicians of notification requirements mandated under contracts.

Law applies to hospital service, medical service, and health service corporations; hospital and medical insurance policies; small employers and individual health benefits plans; and other specified enrollee agreements. In addition, the law directs the State Health Benefits Commission to ensure that every hospital and medical expense benefit plan purchased by the Commission provides the above specified coverage (this provision is effective May 8, 1997).

Law requires state employers covering employees or their family members for the treatment of breast cancer to notify employees as to whether their coverage is subject to the provisions of this law. In addition, the attending physicians of insured patients who will undergo mastectomies or lymph node dissections shall determine if they will be covered under the provisions of the law, and shall notify patients of their findings.

Quality Assurance   Not indicated.

Effective Date   Enacted 1997.

New Mexico   N.M. STAT. ANN. §§ 59A-22-39, 59A-23-4, 59A-23B-3, 59A-46-41

Scope   Reimbursement for Breast Cancer Screening

Woman's Age,   35-39   Baseline
Frequency
of Mammogram   40-49   Every 2 years

                     50+   Each year

Policies   Law requires all health insurance policies to provide coverage for low-dose
and Limits   screening mammograms for determining the presence of breast cancer.

                     The required coverage for mammography *may* be subject to the same deductible
                     and co-insurance requirements as those imposed on other benefits under the same
                     plan.

                     Law applies to individual and group policies, health care plans, certificate of
                     insurance plans, individual and group health maintenance organization policies,
                     and policies that an insurer, fraternal benefit society, health maintenance
                     organization, or nonprofit health care plan offers to individuals, families, or
                     groups of fewer than 20 members pursuant to subsection B of the *Minimum
                     Healthcare Protection Act.* [*See* subsection B for qualifying criteria; N.M. Ann.
                     § 59A-23B-3B].

                     Law does not apply to short-term travel, limited, accident only, or specified
                     disease policies.

                     Law prohibits any blanket or group policy from containing any provision relative
                     to notice or proof of loss or the time for payment of the required benefits.

Quality Assurance After July 1, 1992, the required coverage shall be available only for screening
                     mammograms obtained on equipment designed specifically to perform low-dose
                     mammography in imaging facilities that have met American College of
                     Radiology accreditation standards for mammography.

Effective Date   July 1, 1990; last amended 1993.
                     For policies issued under Subsection B of the Minimum Healthcare Protection
                     Act, 1991. Last amendment effective January 1, 1995.
                     Laws prohibitive of notice, proof of loss, or time limitations in payment of
                     benefits in blanket or group policies, effective July 1, 1992.

New Mexico   N.M. STAT. ANN. § 27-2-12.8

Scope   Reimbursement for Breast Cancer Screening [Medicaid Recipients]

Policies   *Quality Assurance:*
and Limits   Law creates a new section of the Public Assistance Act that shall require the
              Department of Health to ensure that Medicaid patients will not be routinely
              solicited for mammograms and that mammograms they receive will be
              performed based on nationally recognized standards.

              Law mandates that any fee for services made on behalf of the Medicaid
              program for a mammogram received by a Medicaid recipient shall
              be consistent with the usual and customary charge that reflects the fair market
              value of the cost of a mammogram.

Quality Assurance   Not indicated.

Effective Date   Enacted 1997.

New Mexico   N.M. STAT. ANN. §§ 59A-22-39.1, 59A-46-41.1

Scope   Reimbursement for Length of Stay Following Mastectomy

Policies   Law requires all health insurance, health care plans, and health maintenance
and Limits   organizations to provide coverage for a minimum hospital stay of 48 hours
              following a mastectomy and no less than 24 hours following a lymph node
              dissection.

              This law should not be construed to require a minimum length of stay when the
              physician and the patient determine that a shorter stay is appropriate.

              Coverage under these provisions may be subject to deductibles and
              coinsurance consistent with those imposed on other benefits under the same plan
              or policy.

Quality Assurance   Not indicated.

Effective Date   June 20, 1997, 90 days after adjournment of the legislature.

New York   **NY CLS PUB HEALTH §§ 2405 to 2408**

Scope   Breast Cancer Screening and Education Programs

Policies   Law establishes the Breast Cancer Detection and Education Program. The
and Limits   program is established to promote screening and detection of breast cancer
                   among unserved or underserved populations, to educate the public regarding
                   breast cancer and the benefits of early detection, and to provide counseling and
                   referral services.

                   Law directs the Commissioner of Health, in consultation with the Breast Cancer
                   Detection and Education Program Advisory Council, to make grants to approved
                   organizations for the provision of services relating to the screening and detection
                   of breast cancer.

Quality Assurance   Not indicated.

Effective Date   July 10, 1989; last amendment effective July 26, 1995.
                   (Law applicable to Advisory Council under § 2408, effective July 28, 1995).

New York   **NY CLS PUB HEALTH § 2500-C**

Scope   Breast Cancer Screening Program

Policies   Law requires the establishment, promotion, and maintenance of a statewide
and Limits   public information program regarding diethylstilbestrol (DES).

                 Law requires the program to designate and enter into contracts with providers of
                 health care for the purpose of establishing regional screening programs for
                 women who were exposed to DES during pregnancy and their offspring who
                 were exposed prenatally.

                 Law requires consideration of providers' compliance with state and federally
                 mandated standards, the location in relation to the geographic distribution of
                 persons exposed to DES, and the capacity of the provider to properly screen for
                 breast cancer and any other malignancy and abnormal conditions resulting from
                 DES exposure.

                 Law requires the establishment of a program to train physicians, physician's
                 assistants, and nurses in the detection, diagnosis, treatment, and prevention of
                 diseases in women who were exposed to DES during pregnancy and their
                 offspring who were exposed prenatally.

                 Law requires the bureau of cancer control within the health department to
                 establish and maintain a registry of women who took diethylstilbestrol during
                 pregnancy and their offspring who were exposed to diethylstilbestrol prenatally
                 for the purpose of follow-up care and treatment of long-term problems associated
                 with diethylstilbestrol exposure. Enrollment in the registry shall be upon a
                 voluntary basis.

Quality Assurance   Not indicated.

Effective Date   August 7, 1978

New York   NY CLS Ins § 4303(p)

Scope   Reimbursement for Breast Cancer Screening

Woman's Age,   35-39   Baseline
Frequency
of Mammogram   40-49   Every 2 years, or more frequently upon physician's
                                recommendation

                   50+   Each year

                   Any age   Upon physician's recommendation for persons having a prior
                                history of breast cancer or whose mother or sister has a prior
                                history of breast cancer.

                   In no event shall coverage under this law include more than one annual screening.

Policies   Law requires that insurers providing coverage for hospital, medical, or surgical
and Limits   care cover mammography screening for the presence of occult breast cancer.

                   Law applies to medical expense indemnity corporations, hospital service
                   corporations, and health service corporations.

                   Coverage may be subject to annual deductibles and coinsurance consistent with
                   those established for other benefits.

                   Law defines "mammography screening."

Quality Assurance Examination must use dedicated equipment.

Effective Date   January 1, 1990.

New York NY CLS Ins §§ 3216(i)(20), 3221(k)(10), 4303(x)6(I)

Scope Reimbursement for Breast Reconstruction or Prosthesis

Policies Law requires that insurers provide coverage for all stages of reconstruction
and Limits of the removed breast following mastectomy, as well as surgery and
 reconstruction of the other breast to produce a symmetrical appearance in the
 manner deemed appropriate by the physician in consultation with the patient.

 Law applies to all group, blanket, or other policies providing medical, major
 medical, or similar comprehensive coverage; all contracts issued by medical
 indemnity corporations providing coverage for surgical or medical care; and
 contracts issued by medical expense indemnity, health service, or hospital service
 corporations.

 Coverage for breast reconstruction shall be subject to annual deductibles and
 coinsurance deemed appropriate by the Superintendent of Insurance, and as
 consistent with deductible and coinsurance levels established for other benefits
 under the same policy. Insurance plans shall provide written notice of the
 availability of such coverage prior to enacting the policy and annually thereafter.

 Law prohibits insurers providing coverage under this section from denying the
 eligibility of covered persons from enrolling in or renewing their coverage under
 the terms of the policy for the purpose of avoiding compliance with these
 provisions; providing incentives to encourage covered persons to accept less than
 the minimum coverage in these provisions; penalizing health care practitioners
 for providing care consistent with these provisions; and providing incentives for
 health care practitioners to provided care in a manner inconsistent with these
 provisions.

Quality Assurance Not indicated.

Effective Date September 1, 1984; last amendment effective January 1, 1998.

New York   NY PUB HEALTH § 2404 (1-a)

Scope   Alternative Therapies

Policies   Law directs the Commissioner of Health to develop a standardized
and Limits   written summary, in plain non-technical language, that shall explain the
          alternative medically viable methods of treating breast cancer; including,
          but not limited to hormonal, radiological, chemotherapeutic or surgical
          treatments.

          The summary shall also include information on breast reconstructive
          surgery; including but not limited to, the use of breast implants, their side effects,
          risks, and other pertinent information.

          The summary shall also include an explanation of the special provisions relating
          to mastectomy; lymph node dissection, or lumpectomy, breast reconstructive
          surgery; and second-opinion coverage under the insurance law. It shall also
          suggest that patients check with their health plans for details of this coverage.

          The summary shall be provided by physicians to each patient under their care
          who has been diagnosed with breast cancer. The summary shall be updated as
          necessary.

Quality Assurance   Not indicated.

Effective Date   January 1, 1998 (Subsection 1-a was added to § 2404 by amendment in 1997)

New York   **NY Pub Health §§ 2410 to 2413;**
              NY Tax §§ 209-D, 627; NY Fin § 97-yy

Scope   Income Tax Checkoff for Breast Cancer Research

Policies   Law permits taxpayers to contribute to the Breast Cancer Research and
and Limits   Education Fund beginning in 1996. Taxpayers can specify any whole dollar
                contribution on personal or corporate income tax returns. Contributions do not
                reduce the amount of state tax owed by taxpayers.

                In addition to taxpayer contributions, the Breast Cancer Research and Education
                Fund may receive appropriations, grants, gifts, or bequests.

                Law establishes the Health Research Science Board within the Department of
                Health. The Board shall solicit and review applications for grants from the
                Breast Cancer Research and Education Fund. Applications may be submitted by
                public and private agencies and organizations. The Board shall make
                recommendations to the Commissioner of Health, who shall approve applications
                from among those recommended by the Board. The Board shall also identify data
                collected by state agencies that might be of use to breast cancer researchers, and
                shall consult with federal agencies and other organizations involved in cancer
                research to identify current and potential breast cancer research projects.

                Moneys from the Fund can be used only for breast cancer research and education
                projects approved by the Department of Health.

Quality Assurance Not indicated.

Effective Date   Ninety days from October 6, 1996; last amendment effective 180 days from
                   March 26, 2000.

New York   NY CLS INS § 3224

Scope   Restrictions on Denial of Insurance Coverage for Breast Cancer Survivors

Policies   Law states that no insurer shall refuse to issue any policy of life or non-
and Limits   cancelable disability insurance, or cancel or decline to renew such policy because
             an individual has had breast cancer.

             Law only applies if the initial diagnosis of breast cancer has occurred at least 3
             years before the date of application and a physician has certified that the disease
             has not recurred.

             Law does not preclude the establishment of selection criteria based on sound
             underwriting and actuarial principles reasonably related to actual or anticipated
             loss experience.

Quality Assurance   Not indicated.

Effective Date   January 1, 1994.

New York   **NY CLS EDUC § 804**

Scope   Breast Cancer Early Detection Instruction in Public Schools

Policies   Law requires high schools to provide instruction regarding methods of prevention
and Limits   and detection of breast cancer to all students at the senior high school level.

                            Law mandates that such instruction be: (i) an integral part of a required health
                            education course, and (ii) implemented as a continued health guidance (in senior
                            high schools).

Quality Assurance   Law requires teachers to hold certificates in health education.

Effective Date   July 1, 1999 (Subsection 3a was added to § 804 by amendment in 1998).

New York   NY PUB HEALTH §§ 2407, 2409;
                 NY CLS ST FIN § 95-a

Scope   Grant Awards for Breast Cancer Early Detection and Research

Policies   Law establishes the New York State Innovation in Breast Cancer Early Detection
and Limits   and Research Awards Program. The program is created to recognize, reward,
                     and promote innovation in breast cancer prevention, early detection, and
                     research.

                     The program shall be administered by the Breast Cancer Detection and
                     Education Program Advisory Council. The Council shall establish eligibility,
                     nomination, and award criteria and procedures.

                     Awards shall be given annually to health professionals, consumers, nonprofit
                     organizations, or other candidates who, according to the Council, best meet the
                     criteria for receiving awards. All awards must be used by the awardee or their
                     designee for breast cancer prevention, early detection, or research.

                     Awards shall be provided from moneys in the New York State Innovation in
                     Breast Cancer Early Detection and Research Awards Program Fund. The Fund
                     shall consist of moneys appropriated by the state and any grants, gifts, or
                     bequests made to the Council.

Quality Assurance Not indicated.

Effective Date   July 10, 1989; last amendment effective July 26, 1995.

New York   NY INS §§ 3216(I), 3221(k), 4303(v,w);
                        NY PUB HEALTH § 2404(1-a)

Scope   Reimbursement for Inpatient Care Following Treatment for Breast Cancer

Policies   Law requires that insurers who provide coverage for inpatient hospital care
and Limits   following a mastectomy, lymph node dissection, or lumpectomy, provide
                        this coverage for a period of time determined medically appropriate by the
                        attending physician in consultation with the patient.

                        The coverage may be subject to annual deductibles and coinsurance
                        deemed appropriate by the Superintendent of Insurance as they are consistent
                        with deductible and coinsurance levels for other benefits within a given policy.

                        Law prohibits insurers from: providing incentives for covered individuals to
                        accept coverage less than that described above; reducing compensation or
                        otherwise penalizing a health care practitioner for recommending the above care
                        to a patient; providing incentives for a health care practitioner to provide care to
                        a patient that is inconsistent with the above guidelines; or restricting coverage for
                        any portion of a hospital stay in a manner that is inconsistent with the coverage
                        provided for any preceding portion of the stay.

                        In addition, physicians are required to provide information about special
                        coverage provisions for mastectomy, lymph node dissection, lumpectomy, and
                        breast reconstructive surgery coverage to patients, and to suggest that patients
                        undergoing these procedures check with their health plans and/or insurance
                        policies for exact details about the coverage to which they are entitled.

Quality Assurance   Not indicated.

Effective Date   September 1, 1984; last amendment effective January 1, 1998.
                        [NY CLS Pub Health § 2404 (1-a), effective January 1, 1998.]

New York   **NY CLS Veh & Tr § 404-q**

Scope   Special License Plates Supporting Breast Cancer Research and Education

Policies   Law authorizes the issuance of distinctive "Drive for the Cure" license plates in
and Limits   support of breast, prostate and testicular cancer research bearing the phrase
                      "Drive for the Cure."

                      Law states that the distinctive plates shall be issued in the same manner as other
                      number plates upon the payment of the regular registration fee and an additional
                      annual service charge of $25 to be charged for the license plate. Fifty percent of
                      the annual service charges shall be deposited to the credit of the Breast Cancer
                      Research and Education Fund and shall be used for research and education
                      programs.

Quality Assurance   Not indicated.

Effective Date   March 26, 2000.

North Carolina   N.C. GEN. STAT. §§ 58-50-155(a), 58-51-57, 58-65-92, 58-67-76

Scope	Reimbursement for Breast Cancer Screening	
Woman's Age, Frequency of Mammogram	35-39	Baseline
	40-49	Every other year, or more frequently upon physician's recommendation
	50+	Each year
	Any age	One or more mammograms a year, upon physician's recommendation for any woman who is at risk for breast cancer (having a personal history of breast cancer; having a personal history of biopsy-proven benign breast disease; whose mother, sister, or daughter has or has had breast cancer; or has not given birth before age 30).

Policies and Limits

Law requires that insurers provide coverage for low-dose screening mammography.

Law applies to accident or health insurance policies or contracts; preferred provider contracts; hospital service plan or medical service plan certificates or contracts; and health maintenance organization plans.

The same deductibles, coinsurance, and other limitations as apply to similar services covered under the policy, contract, or plan apply.

Screening includes a physician's interpretation of the results of the procedures.

Law defines "low-dose mammography screening."

Quality Assurance   Screening must use equipment dedicated specifically for mammography.

Effective Date   January 1, 1992; last amendment effective January 1, 1998.

North Carolina   N.C. GEN. STAT. §§ 135-40.5(e), 135-40.6(8)(s)

Scope   Reimbursement for Breast Cancer Screening for Public Employees

Woman's Age,   -40   Every 3 years
Frequency
of Mammogram   40-49   Every 2 years

   50+   Each year, or more frequently if medically necessary.

Policies   Law requires that the teachers', state employees', and social security health
and Limits   benefit plans pay 100 percent of allowable charges for clinical breast
   examinations and mammograms (and other routine diagnostic examinations, up
   to a maximum of $150 per fiscal year per covered individual). The schedule
   shown above applies unless more frequent examinations are warranted by a
   medical condition and the additional examinations are performed in a medically
   supervised facility.

   Examinations are not covered when they are incurred to obtain or continue
   employment, to secure insurance coverage, to comply with legal proceedings, to
   attend schools or camps, to meet travel requirements, to participate in athletic
   and related activities, or to comply with governmental licensing requirements.

Quality Assurance   Not indicated.

Effective Date   Enacted 1982; last amended 1995.

North Carolina   N.C. GEN STAT. §§ 58-51-62, 58-65-96,
                      58-67-79, 58-50-155, 135-40.6(5)

Scope   Reimbursement for Breast Reconstruction and Prosthesis

Policies   Law requires every health insurance policy that provides coverage for
and Limits   mastectomy also provide coverage for reconstructive breast surgery, prosthesis,
                       and physical complications in all stages of the mastectomy, including
                       lymphademas.

                       Law mandates that the required coverage include coverage for all stages and
                       revisions of reconstructive breast surgery performed on a nondiseased breast to
                       establish symmetry (if reconstructive surgery has been performed on a diseased
                       breast).

                       Law requires that following mastectomy, reconstruction of the nipple/areolar
                       complex be covered, without regard for lapse of time between the mastectomy
                       and reconstruction, subject to approval of the insured's treating physician.

                       Law applies to every policy of accident and health insurance; preferred provider
                       benefit plan; insurance certificate; subscriber contract under any hospital service
                       plan or medical service plan; and health care plan written by a health
                       maintenance organization.

                       Law applies to all such policies in force, issued, renewed, or amended on or after
                       January 1, 1998.

                       Law requires the insurer to provide and deliver to every insured individual, upon
                       initial coverage under the respective policy and annually thereafter, written notice
                       of the availability of the required coverage (effective July 22, 1999).

                       Law prohibits health insurance providers and policy provisions from denying
                       anyone eligibility, eligibility to enroll, eligibility to renew coverage, or, under a
                       policy still in effect, the required coverage: (i) on the basis that the coverage is
                       for cosmetic surgery; (ii) solely for the purpose of avoiding the requirement of
                       the law; (iii) by providing monetary payments or rebates to a woman to
                       encourage her to accept less than the minimum protections available under the
                       law; (iv) penalize or otherwise reduce or limit the reimbursement of an attending
                       medical provider for providing care consistent with these provisions; and (v)
                       provide incentives, monetary or otherwise, to an attending medical provider
                       because he or she gave care to an insured individual in a manner consistent with
                       the law.

The same deductibles, coinsurance, and other limitations as apply to similar services under the respective policy shall apply for reconstructive breast surgery. *(Note: Here, the law states only "reconstructive breast surgery". Law omits any reference concerning the applicability of this specific provision in the law to its required coverage for prosthesis or physical complications following mastectomy).*

Law does not apply to policies for specified accident or disease, hospital indemnity, or long-term care health insurance policies.

Law defines "mastectomy" and "reconstructive breast surgery."

Quality Assurance   Not indicated.

Effective Date   January 1, 1998; last amendment effective July 22, 1999.

North Carolina   N.C. Gen. Stat. § 58-3-168

Scope

Reimbursement for Inpatient Care Following Mastectomy

*Policies
and Limits*

Law requires health benefit plans providing coverage for mastectomy to ensure that decisions about whether to discharge a patient following this procedure are made by the attending physician in consultation with the patient, and that the decision is based on the unique characteristics and medical history of the patient.

Law applies to individual and group accident and health insurance policies or certificates; nonprofit hospital or medical service corporation contracts; health, hospital, or medical service corporation plan contracts; health maintenance organization (HMO) subscriber contracts; and plans provided by a MEWA or plans provided by other benefit arrangements.

Law defines "mastectomy."

Quality Assurance

Not indicated.

Effective Date

August 28, 1997; enacted as § 58-3-171.1, was then codified as this section

North Dakota   N.D. Cen. Code § 26.1-36-09.1

Scope   Reimbursement for Breast Cancer Screening

Woman's Age,   35-39   Baseline
Frequency
of Mammogram   40-49   Every 2 years, or more frequently upon physician's order

   50+   Each year

Policies   Law requires that insurers provide mammogram examination coverage.
and Limits

   Law applies to insurance companies, nonprofit health service corporations, and health maintenance organizations.

   Law does not apply to individually guaranteed renewable supplemental, specified disease, long-term care, or other limited benefit policies.

Quality Assurance   Not indicated.

Effective Date   July 1, 1989.

Ohio　　　　　　　**ORC Ann. § 5.2213**

Scope　　　　　　Breast Cancer Education Programs

Policies　　　　　Law designates the month of October as "Ohio Breast Cancer Awareness
and Limits　　　　Month," and the third Thursday of each October as "Ohio Mammography Day,"
　　　　　　　　　to promote the importance of identifying breast cancer in its earliest stages.

Quality Assurance　Not indicated.

Effective Date　　May 21, 1998

Ohio   ORC ANN. §§ 1742.40, 1751.62, 3923.52 to 3923.54, 5111.024

Scope   Reimbursement for Breast Cancer Screening

Woman's Age,   35-39   Baseline
Frequency
of Mammogram   40-49   Every 2 years, but every year if physician determines that the
                                  women has risk factors for breast cancer

                    50-64   Each year

Policies   Law requires every health insurance policy to provide screening mammography
and Limits   benefits for the purpose of detecting the presence of breast cancer in adult
                            women.

                            Law applies to every health insurance policy of individual or group sickness and
                            accident, including employee, public employee (provided in whole or in part), and
                            health care benefit plans; individual or group health insuring corporate policy
                            providing basic health care services; and, public welfare medical assistance
                            program health care policies.

                            Law does not apply to any policy that provides coverage for specific diseases or
                            accidents only, or to any hospital indemnity, medicare supplement, or other
                            policy that offers only supplemental benefits.

                            Required Benefit Limits:
                            The screening mammography benefits required under this law shall not exceed
                            $85 per year, unless a lower amount is established pursuant to the inspection
                            policy *if* the policy is one of individual or group health sickness and accident;
                            public employee health care benefit plan; or, individual or group health insuring
                            corporate policy.

                            Screening mammography benefits required under this law need not exceed $85
                            per year (and are not subject to policy provisions establishing a lower amount) if
                            the policy is an employee health care benefits plan (provided in whole or in part)
                            under a policy of sickness and accident insurance.

Benefits paid under this law constitutes full payment. Law prohibits any further compensation to the provider.

The screening mammography benefits required by this law shall be included in public welfare medical assistance policies only: (i) if federal approval is received, and (ii) approval for use of federal funds is granted to the state's public welfare department.

Law defines "screening mammography" to include the professional interpretation of the film, and to exclude diagnostic mammography.

Quality Assurance   Examination must use equipment dedicated specifically for mammography.

Facility must be accredited under the American College of Radiology Mammography Accreditation Program.

Effective Date   July 1, 1992; last amendment effective March 22, 1999. [Law applicable to policies issued under public welfare medical assistance programs first became effective July 1, 1992; last amendment effective November 24, 1995]

Oklahoma   **63 OKL. ST. §§ 1-554 TO 1-558**

Scope   Breast Cancer Screening and Education Programs/
                     Income Tax Checkoff for Breast Cancer Screening and Research

Policies   Law creates the Oklahoma Breast Cancer Prevention and Treatment Advisory
and Limits   Committee within the Oklahoma Center for the Advancement of Science and
                     Technology. The Committee shall advise the Center on contracting for statewide
                     breast cancer screening and education services. These services shall include
                     mammography screening, referral for definitive diagnosis, education and training
                     programs for health care professionals, annual public education awareness
                     campaigns, epidemiological trend studies, and outreach to uninsured and
                     underinsured groups.

                     Each year, the Committee shall report to the Governor and the Legislature on the
                     breast cancer screening and education services.

                     Law establishes the Breast Cancer Act Revolving Fund. Checkoffs are created on
                     individual and corporate state income tax returns permitting taxpayers to
                     contribute amounts from their tax refunds to the Fund. Moneys in the Fund may
                     be used for the statewide breast cancer screening and education services, or
                     transferred to the Research Support Revolving Fund to support breast cancer
                     research. Moneys may also be expended for promotional activities to encourage
                     donations to the Fund.

                     Payments for breast cancer screening shall be at the accepted Medicare/Medicaid
                     rate and a sliding fee schedule shall be employed to encourage self-responsibility.

Quality Assurance Mammography screening shall be provided by facilities accredited by national
                     organizations that have formed coalitions to issue national cancer screening
                     guidelines.

Effective Date   July 1, 1994; amended November 1, 1995, and May 7, 1996.

Oklahoma 36 OKL. ST. § 6060

Scope   Reimbursement for Breast Cancer Screening

Woman's Age,   35-39   Baseline
Frequency
of Mammogram   40+   Each year

                     [Prior law, effective November 1, 1988, required mammography coverage for
                     women, age 45 and older]

Policies   Law requires that individual and group health insurance policies providing
and Limits   coverage on an expense-incurred basis and all individual and group service or
                     indemnity type contracts issued by nonprofit corporations and self-insurers
                     include coverage for low-dose mammography for the presence of occult breast
                     cancer.

                     Law does not apply to policies that provide specified disease or other limited
                     benefit coverage.

                     Law limits reimbursement to $75.

                     Law defines "low-dose mammography."

Quality Assurance Examination must use equipment dedicated specifically for mammography.

Effective Date   November 1, 1989.

Oklahoma   **36 OKL. St. § 6060.5**

Scope   Reimbursement for Breast Reconstruction and Prosthesis

Policies and Limits   Law establishes the Oklahoma Breast Cancer Patient Protection Act. It requires that all health benefit plans that provide medical or surgical benefits with respect to breast cancer or other breast conditions shall provide coverage for reconstructive breast surgery following a mastectomy. This surgery shall include reconstruction of the diseased breast as well as reconstructive surgery performed on the non-diseased breast to achieve symmetry. Coverage is contingent upon the surgery on the non-diseased breast being performed within 24 months of surgery on the diseased breast.

The insurer may not modify the terms of coverage based on the determination by an enrollee to request less than the minimum coverage described above.

Law requires health benefit plans to notify all enrollees of the coverage provided in this law no later than December 1, 1997.

Quality Assurance   Not indicated.

Effective Date   November 1, 1997.

Oklahoma   **36 OKL. ST. § 6060**.5

Scope   Reimbursement for Inpatient Care Following Mastectomy

Policies and   Law establishes the Oklahoma Breast Cancer Patient Protection Act. It requires
Limits   that all health benefit plans that provide medical or surgical
                     benefits with respect to breast cancer or other breast conditions shall
                     ensure that coverage is provided for not less than 48 hours following a
                     mastectomy and for not less than 24 hours following a lymph node
                     dissection.

                     Law should not be construed as requiring a minimum length of stay if the
                     physician, in consultation with the patient, has determined a shorter
                     length of stay to be appropriate. The insurer may not modify the terms of
                     coverage based on the determination by an enrollee to request less than
                     the minimum coverage as described above.

                     Law requires health benefit plans to notify all enrollees of the coverage provided
                     in this law no later than December 1, 1997.

Quality Assurance Not indicated.

Effective Date   November 1, 1997.

Oklahoma   **47 OKL. St. § 1136**

Scope   Special License Plates Supporting Breast Cancer Screening and Research

Policies   Law authorizes the Oklahoma Tax Commission to design and issue special motor
and Limits   vehicle license plates recognizing a variety of groups and causes. Among the
                   special plates authorized is one bearing the legend "Fight Breast Cancer."

                   This plate can be obtained for $25 to demonstrate support for the prevention and
                   treatment of breast cancer in Oklahoma. The Breast Cancer Act Revolving Fund
                   (see page 169, Breast Cancer Screening and Education Programs) shall receive
                   $20 from each plate sold; the Fund supports breast cancer screening, education,
                   and research programs.

Quality Assurance   Not indicated.

Effective Date   November 1, 1996.

Oklahoma   63 OKL. ST. § 1-743

Scope   Advertising of Mammography Services

Policies   Law requires that advertising for mammography services include the
and Limits   total cost of the procedure.

Quality Assurance   Not indicated.

Effective Date   September 1, 1993.

Oregon   **ORS § 743.727**

Scope   Reimbursement for Breast Cancer Screening

Woman's Age,   40+   Each year, with or without referral from health care provider
Frequency
of Mammogram   Any age   Upon referral from health care provider for women who are
                                  symptomatic or at high-risk for breast cancer

Policies   Law requires insurers to offer coverage for screening and diagnostic
and Limits   mammography.

                       Law applies to health insurance policies that cover hospital, medical or surgical
                       expenses.

                       Law does not apply to supplemental contracts covering a specified disease or
                       other limited benefits.

Quality Assurance   Not indicated.

Effective Date   1993; last amendment effective July 1, 1999

Pennsylvania 40 P.S. § 764c

Scope	Reimbursement for Breast Cancer Screening

Woman's Age, Frequency of Mammogram	-40	Upon physician's recommendation
	40+	Each year

[Prior law, effective July 7, 1989, required mammography coverage for women aged 50 and older]

Policies and Limits

Law requires that insurers provide coverage for mammographic examinations.

Law applies to group or individual health or sickness or accident policies providing hospital or medical/surgical coverage; hospital plan corporation and professional health service plan corporation group or individual subscriber contracts or certificates; health maintenance organizations; fraternal benefit societies; and ERISA employee welfare benefit plans.

Law does not require an insurer to cover mastectomies and does not prevent the application of deductible or copayment provisions contained in the policy or plan.

Quality Assurance

Prior to payment, insurers shall verify that the screening mammography service provider is properly licensed under the Mammography Quality Assurance Act.[*]

Effective Date

Sixty days after December 15, 1992.

NOTE: 1994 Laws, Act 20, the Women's Preventative Health Services Act, effective 60 days after April 22, 1994, requires that health insurance policies include coverage for annual clinical breast examinations. The law provides for the repeal of all previous acts inconsistent with the 1994 enactment.

Pennsylvania   **1997 Pₐ. ALS 51; 1997 Pₐ. SB 176**

Scope   Reimbursement for Length of Stay/Inpatient Care Following Mastectomy
                       Reimbursement for Breast Reconstruction and Prosthesis

Policies   Law amends the Insurance Company Law of 1921 (P.L. 682, No. 284) to require
and Limits   health insurance policies to provide coverage of inpatient care following a
                       mastectomy for the length of stay deemed necessary by the physician for meeting
                       the criteria for a safe discharge.

                       Law also provides for a home health care visit that the physician deems
                       necessary within 48 hours after hospital discharge when the discharge occurs
                       within 48 hours following hospital admission for the procedure.

                       Law requires policies that cover mastectomy to also provide coverage for
                       prosthetic devices and reconstructive surgery incident to the mastectomy.

                       Coverage under this section shall be subject to all policy copayment,
                       coinsurance, and deductible amounts. Coverage for services incident to
                       mastectomy may be limited to procedures performed within six years of the date
                       of the mastectomy.

                       Law does not apply to policies limited to accident only, credit, dental, specified
                       disease, or other limited benefit plans.

                       Law defines the following terms: mastectomy, prosthetic devices, reconstructive
                       surgery, and symmetry between breasts.

Quality Assurance   Not indicated.

Effective Date   January 1, 1998.

Pennsylvania   35 P.S. §§ 5651 to 5664

Scope   Accreditation of Facilities and Technologists

Policies   Law requires that a radiation machine used for mammography have authorization
and Limits   from the Pennsylvania Department of Health. Licenses to operate radiation
machines are effective for 3 years and are based on meeting the following
criteria:

\# The radiation machine meets the criteria established by regulations issued
under the Omnibus Budget Reconciliation Act of 1990 (OBRA).

\# The radiation machine is specifically designed for mammography.

\# The provider of mammography screening, in accordance with criteria
established by regulations issued under OBRA, establishes a quality control
program, including inspections by a qualified radiation physicist and retains and
makes available to patients the original mammograms.

\# A radiation technologist who meets criteria established by regulations issued
under OBRA operates the radiation machine.

\# The interpreting physician meets the criteria established by regulations issued
under OBRA.

The law provides for application procedures, initial and annual inspections by the
Department, suspensions or revocations, nonrenewals, provider violations, fees,
and regulations.

Effective Date   Sixty days from July 9, 1992.

Pennsylvania   **35 P.S. §§ 5641, 5642**

Scope   Alternative Therapies/Informed Consent for Treatment of Breast Cancer

Policies and   Law requires the execution of a consent form before a physician operates on a
Limits   patient for a breast tumor. Failure to comply with this law subjects the physician
to civil liability in addition to disciplinary action under the appropriate licensing
act.

The consent form must include the following:

"CONSENT FOR TREATMENT OF BREAST DISEASE"

Sign option (a) or option (b), or option (a) and option (b).

(a) ....Breast Biopsy
Side (right or left)

....
Patient's Signature

(b) If it is determined that I have a malignant tumor in my breast or other breast
abnormality requiring surgery, then I authorize Dr.................... to perform such
operations or procedures, including breast removal, which are deemed necessary.
I have been informed of the current medically accepted alternatives to radical
mastectomy.

Procedure:
....
....
Patient's Signature

Quality Assurance   Not indicated.

Effective Date   Sixty days from December 18, 1984.

Pennsylvania   **72 P.S. § 7315.2**

Scope   Income Tax Checkoff for Breast Cancer Research

Policies and   Law creates an income tax checkoff to allow a contribution to breast cancer
Limits   research. Directs the Department of Revenue to create the space for this checkoff
                     and to provide adequate instructions within the tax form to include information
                     about the use of the funds. Law directs the Department of Health to conduct a
                     public information campaign to make taxpayers aware of the opportunity to
                     contribute in this manner.

                     Funds will go to the Pennsylvania Cancer Control, Prevention, and Research
                     Advisory Board within the Department of Health.

Quality Assurance Not indicated.

Effective Date   Enacted upon passage, May 7, 1997.

Rhode Island   **R.I. GEN. LAWS §§ 27-18-41 to 27-18-42, 27-19-20, 27-20-17, 27-41-31, 42-62-26**

Scope   Reimbursement for Breast Cancer Screening

Woman's Age,   Not stipulated.
Frequency
of Mammogram

Policies   Law requires insurance coverage for mammograms in accordance with
and Limits   American Cancer Society guidelines.

   Law applies to insurers, nonprofit hospital service plans, nonprofit
   medical service plans, and health maintenance organizations.

   Law does not apply to insurance companies providing benefits for hospital
   confinement indemnity; disability income; accident only; long-term care;
   Medicare supplement; limited benefit health; specified disease indemnity;
   sickness or bodily injury or death by accident or both; and other limited benefit
   policies.

Quality Assurance   Mammograms will be eligible for reimbursement only if the facility in which the
   mammogram is performed and processed and the physician interpreting the
   mammogram meet state-approved quality assurance standards.

Effective Date   1988 (Coverage); 1989 (Quality Assurance)

Rhode Island   **R.I. GEN. LAWS §§ 27-18-39, 27-19-34, 27-20-21, 27-20-29, 27-41-43**

Scope   Reimbursement for Breast Reconstruction and Prosthesis

Policies   Law requires insurers to cover prosthetic devices and/or reconstructive surgery
and Limits   incident to a mastectomy, but does not require coverage of mastectomies. The
     reconstructive surgery must be performed within 18 months of the mastectomy.

     Law applies to individual and group accident and sickness insurance
     policies; individual and group contracts, plans, or policies issued by
     nonprofit hospital or medical service corporations; and health maintenance
     organizations. To be subject to the law, however, such policies must
     cover physician services delivered in a physician's office or provide
     major medical or similar comprehensive coverage. Policies that only
     cover specified diseases and other supplemental policies are exempt.

     The mandated coverage shall be subject to the deductible and coinsurance
     conditions applied to the mastectomy as well as to all other terms and conditions
     of the policy. Managed care and medical necessity reviews
     by an insurer are allowed.

     Law defines "prosthetic devices" and "mastectomy."

Quality Assurance   Not indicated.

Effective Date   January 1, 1997.

Rhode Island   **R.I. GEN. LAWS §§ 5-37-31, 23-17-32, 27-19-21, 27-20-18, 27-41-30, 42-62-27**

Scope   Accreditation of Facilities and Technologists

Policies   Law requires that any licensed facility performing a mammogram meet
and Limits   state-approved quality assurance standards for taking and processing
                 mammograms.

                 Any licensed physician interpreting a mammogram shall meet
                 state-approved quality assurance standards.

                 The law authorizes the Rhode Island Director of Health to issue necessary rules
                 and regulations.

Effective Date September 1, 1989.

Scope   Fund for Breast Cancer Screening, Research and Treatment

Policies   Law establishes the Rhode Island Research and Treatment Fund for Breast and
and Limits   Cervical Cancer. The General Treasurer is authorized to accept any grant,
                         devise, bequest, donation, gift, services in kind, or assignment of money, bonds,
                         or other valuable securities for deposit in the Fund.

                         Annually, by September 30, the state shall equally distribute the moneys in the
                         Fund to all organizations that have been certified by the Department of Health
                         for the funding year. All funds distributed must be used for research on the
                         prevention of breast or cervical cancer, or for the diagnosis and treatment of
                         breast and cervical cancers among uninsured or underinsured women. The funds
                         shall be supplemental to all other moneys available for these purposes.

                         Eligible organizations that seek to qualify for funds must submit an application
                         to the Department of Health not later than July 15 of each year.

Quality Assurance   Not indicated.

Effective Date   1995; reenacted and recodified 1997.

Rhode Island   **R.I. GEN. LAWS §§ 27-18-40, 27-19-34.1, 27-20-29.1,
                      27-41-43.1**

Scope   Reimbursement for Inpatient Care Following Mastectomy

Policies   Law requires insurers to cover a minimum 48-hour inpatient stay in a
and Limits   hospital following mastectomy and a minimum 24-hour stay after an
                      axillary node dissection. Any decision to shorten these minimum coverages shall
                      be made by the attending physician in consultation with the patient.
                      If a shorter stay is authorized, insurers shall cover a minimum of one
                      home visit conducted by a physician or registered nurse.

                      Law provides penalties for plans that do not cover the benefits outlined
                      above, and no plan may terminate the services, reduce capitated
                      payment, or otherwise penalize an attending physician or other health care
                      provider who orders care consistent with these benefits. In addition, it requires
                      plans to provide notice of these benefits to enrollees.

                      Law does not apply to hospital confinement indemnity, accident only,
                      long- term care, and other supplemental plans providing limited benefits.
                      The mandated coverage shall be subject to the deductible and coinsurance
                      conditions applied to the mastectomy as well as to all other terms and conditions
                      of the policy.

Quality Assurance   Not indicated.

Effective Date   Upon passage, June 10, 1997.

South Carolina   S.C. CODE ANN. § 38-71-145

Scope   Reimbursement for Breast Cancer Screening

Woman's Age,   35-39   Baseline
Frequency
of Mammogram   40-49   Every 2 years

                        50+   Each year

Policies and Limits   Law requires every health insurance policy to provide coverage for mammography screening made in accordance with the minimum frequency specified above and with the most recent published guidelines of the American Cancer Society.

                        Law applies to all individual, group health insurance policies by a fraternal benefit society, an insurer, a health maintenance organization, or any similar entity (except as exempted by ERISA).

                        Law prohibits the required coverage from including any exclusion, reduction, or other limitations as to such coverage, deductibles, or coinsurance provisions that apply unless the prohibited provision(s) apply generally to other similar benefits provided and paid for under the respective policy.

                        Nothing in the law prohibits any such policy from providing benefits *greater* than those required by this law.

                        Law defines "mammogram" and "health insurance policy."

Quality Assurance   Facilities must utilize radiological equipment approved by the Department of Health and Environmental Control.

Effective Date   June 8, 1998.

South Carolina   S.C. CODE ANN. § 38-71-130

Scope

Reimbursement for Breast Reconstruction and Prosthesis

Policies and Limits

Law requires every health insurance policy that provides coverage for mastectomy to also provide coverage for reconstructive breast surgery and prosthetic devices.

Law mandates that the required coverage include coverage for surgery and reconstruction of the non-diseased breast, if determined medically necessary by the patient's attending physician, with approval of the insurer or health maintenance organization. *(The provisions of this law do not require supplemental health insurance policies to provide coverage for reconstruction of the non-diseased breast.)*

Law applies to all individual, group health insurance policies and health maintenance organization policies issued, delivered, issued for delivery, or renewed in the state of South Carolina on or after January 1, 1999.

Quality Assurance

Not indicated.

Effective Date

January 1, 1999.

South Carolina   S.C. CODE ANN. § 38-71-125

Scope   Reimbursement for Inpatient Stay Following Mastectomy

Policies   Part of the Omnibus Health Benefits and Education Act of 1998,
and Limits   amending the Code of Laws of South Carolina, 1976. Requires that all
                     individual and group insurance policies and health maintenance
                     organizations providing coverage for the hospitalization for mastectomies must
                     provide benefits for hospitalization for at least 48 hours following a mastectomy.

                     Law should not be construed to prohibit an attending physician from
                     releasing a patient prior to 48 hours following the mastectomy. In the
                     case of an early release, coverage shall include at least one home care
                     visit if ordered by the attending physician.

                     Applies to insurance policies issued, delivered, issued for delivery, or renewed in
                     the state on or after January 1, 1999.

Quality Assurance Not indicated.

Effective Date   January 1, 1999.

Scope   Breast Cancer Screening and Education Programs

Policies and   Law states that the South Dakota Department of Health may establish a program
Limits   to provide education to the public on mammograms.

                        The Department may establish a program to provide money to medical
                        institutions for mammograms. The grant program shall subsidize mammograms
                        based upon the recipient's income.

                        Institutions receiving grants must report on the frequency of mammogram, the
                        amount of subsidies provided, and the detection of cancer resulting from those
                        mammograms.

Quality Assurance   Not indicated.

Effective Date   July 1, 1991.

South Dakota   S.D. CODIFIED LAWS §§ 58-17-1.1, 58-18-36, 58-38-22,
                     58-40-20, 58-41-35.5

Scope   Reimbursement for Breast Cancer Screening

Woman's Age,   35-39   Baseline
Frequency
of Mammogram   40-49   Every 2 years

                     50+   Each year

Policies   Law requires that insurers provide coverage for low-dose screening
and Limits   mammography.

                     Law applies to health insurance policies; group health insurance policies; service
                     or indemnity-type contracts issued by nonprofit medical and surgical service plan
                     corporations and nonprofit hospital service plan corporations;
                     and health maintenance organization contracts.

                     Law does not apply to policies that provide coverage for specified disease or
                     other limited benefit coverage.

                     Law defines "low-dose screening mammography."

Quality Assurance Equipment must be dedicated specifically for mammography.

Effective Date   July 1, 1990.

Tennessee   TENN. CODE ANN. §§ 56-7-1012, 56-7-2502

Scope   Reimbursement for Breast Cancer Screening

Woman's Age,   35-39   Baseline
Frequency
of Mammogram   40-49   Every 2 years, or more frequently upon physician's
                              recommendation

                     50+   Each year

                     Physician referral required.

Policies   Law requires that insurers providing coverage for surgical services for
and Limits   mastectomy also provide coverage for mammography screening.

                     Law applies to individual, franchise, blanket, or group health insurance policies;
                     medical service plans; hospital service corporation contracts; hospital and
                     medical service corporation contracts; fraternal benefit societies; and health
                     maintenance organizations.

                     Law also applies to insurance policies providing benefits only for specified
                     disease if the policies cover mastectomies, unless the policy owner has other
                     insurance covering mammography. The issuer of a specified disease policy has
                     the burden of proving the insured has other insurance that covers mammography.

                     Law does not apply to Medicare supplemental policies unless mammography is
                     covered under Medicare.

                     Law does not apply to policies providing only hospital indemnity benefits or to
                     policies providing only benefits for specified accidents.

Quality Assurance Examination must be performed on dedicated equipment.

Effective Date   July 1, 1989.

Tennessee　　　**TENN. CODE ANN. § 56-7-2507**

Scope　　　　　Reimbursement for Breast Reconstruction and Prosthesis

Policies　　　　Law requires that insurers that provide benefits for mastectomy also provide
and Limits　　coverage for all stages of reconstructive breast surgery on the diseased breast as
　　　　　　　a result of mastectomy, as well as any surgical procedure on the non-diseased
　　　　　　　breast deemed necessary to establish symmetry between the two breasts in the
　　　　　　　manner chosen by the physician. The surgical procedure performed on the non-
　　　　　　　diseased breast must occur within 5 years of the date of the surgery performed on
　　　　　　　the diseased breast.

　　　　　　　Benefits do not apply to reconstructive surgery following a lumpectomy.

　　　　　　　Coverage for reconstructive breast surgery shall be subject to applicable
　　　　　　　copayments, coinsurance, and deductibles.

Quality Assurance　Not indicated.

Effective Date　　July 1, 1997.

Tennessee   TENN. CODE ANN. § 56-7-2504

Scope   Reimbursement for Chemotherapy and Bone Marrow Transplant
                     for Breast Cancer

Policies   Law requires insurers to provide coverage for the treatment of cancer by dose-
and Limits   intensive chemotherapy/autologous bone marrow transplants or stem cell
                     transplants. However, this requirement applies only in the event that such
                     coverage is instituted for enrollees in TennCare (the state Medicaid program).

                     The mandate, if applied, pertains to individual or group accident and sickness
                     insurance policies providing hospital, medical/surgical, or major medical
                     coverage on an expense-incurred basis; individual or group accident and sickness
                     subscription contracts; and health care plans provided by health maintenance
                     organizations. Exempted are short-term travel, long-term care, credit, dental,
                     disability income, medical/surgical supplemental, vision, hospital indemnity, and
                     accident-only insurance; limited or specified-disease policies; and short-term
                     nonrenewable policies of not more than six months duration.

                     The coverage may be offered at an additional cost, but any deductibles shall not
                     be greater than any other deductibles in the policy, and any copayment shall not
                     exceed the standard copayment required in the policy.

Quality Assurance Not indicated.

Effective Date   January 1, 1996.

| Texas | TEX. HEALTH & SAFETY CODE §§ 86.001 to 86.005 |

Scope   Breast Cancer Screening and Education Programs/Alternative Therapies

Policies   Law directs the Texas Department of Health to publish a standardized
and Limits   written summary, in language a patient can understand, of the advantages,
disadvantages, risks, and descriptions of all medically efficacious and viable
alternatives for breast cancer treatment.

The Department shall update the summary annually if necessary. An
advisory council shall develop the summary.

The Department shall make sufficient copies of the summary available to all
physicians in the state. A physician may distribute the summary to a patient
when the physician's professional judgment determines it is in the patient's best
interest.

Quality Assurance   Not indicated.

Effective Date   September 1, 1991.

Texas   TEX. HEALTH & SAFETY CODE §§ 86.011 to 86.012

Scope   Breast Cancer Screening and Education Programs

Policies   Law states that the Texas Center for Rural Health Initiatives, in coordination
and Limits   with the Texas Cancer Council, may provide breast cancer screening in counties
                           with populations of 50,000 or less.

                           The Center may contract with public or private entities for screening.

                           The Center may appoint an advisory committee to advise the Office of Rural
                           Health on breast cancer screening.

Quality Assurance   Not indicated.

Effective Date   September 1, 1991.

Texas   TEX. INS. CODE ART. 3.70-2(H), 3.74(3A)

Scope   Reimbursement for Breast Cancer Screening

Woman's Age,   35+Each year
Frequency
of Mammogram

Policies   Law requires that individual or group policy of accident and sickness insurance
and Limits   and Medicare supplement policies include coverage for
screening by low-dose mammography for the presence of occult breast cancer.

Law does not apply to policies that provide coverage for specified disease
or other limited benefit coverage.

Coverage may not be less favorable than for other radiological
examinations and is subject to the same dollar limits, deductibles, and
coinsurance factors.

Quality Assurance   Examination must be performed on equipment dedicated specifically for
mammography.

Effective Date   September 1, 1987.

Texas TEX. INS. CODE ART. 21.53D

Scope Reimbursement for Breast Reconstruction

Policies Law requires health benefit plans that provide coverage for mastectomies to also
and Limits provide coverage for breast reconstruction.

Law applies to health benefit plans that provide benefits for medical or surgical
expenses incurred as a result of a health condition, accident, or sickness,
including: an individual, group, blanket, or franchise insurance policy or
agreement, or a group hospital service contract. Law also applies to an individual
or group evidence of coverage that is offered by: an insurance company; a group
hospital service corporation, a fraternal benefit society; a stipulated premium
insurance company; and a health maintenance organization.

Law also applies to health benefit plans that provide coverage only for a specific
disease or condition or for hospitalization.

Law does not apply to plans that provide coverage: (i) only for accidental death
or dismemberment; (ii) for wages or payments in lieu of wages for a period
during which an employee is absent from work because of sickness or injury; or
(iii) as a supplement to liability insurance. Law also does not apply to Medicare
supplemental policies, workers' compensation policies, medical payment
insurance issued as part of motor vehicle insurance policies, or long-term care
policies.

Law prohibits insurers to offer any financial incentives for a patient to forgo
breast reconstruction or to waive the coverage required by this law.

Law defines "breast reconstruction."

Quality Assurance Not indicated.

Effective Date September 1, 1997.

Texas   TEX. HEALTH & SAFETY CODE §§ 401.421 to 401.431

Scope   Accreditation of Facilities

Policies   Law requires certification of mammography systems. Certification is valid for
and Limits   one year.

                             The Department shall apply under the Mammography Quality Standards
                             Act of 1992 to become an accreditation body and carry out certification program
                             requirements and to implement standards of the U.S. Secretary of Health under
                             that Act.

                             To receive a mammography certification the mammography system must,
                             at a minimum:

                             # meet criteria as stringent as those of the American College of Radiology
                             Mammography Accreditation Program;

                             # be specifically designed and used for mammography;

                             # be operated by a certified medical radiologic technologist who meets, at a
                             minimum, the requirements for personnel who perform mammography
                             established by the Mammography Quality Standards Act of 1992; and

                             # be used in a facility that meets certification requirements under Mammography
                             Quality Standards Act of 1992, has a licensed medical physicist provide annual
                             on-site consultation, has a quality control program that meets requirements as
                             stringent as those of the American College of Radiology Mammography
                             Accreditation Program, and satisfies specified record keeping requirements.

                             The Board may accept certification by the American College of Radiology or
                             other recognized organization.

                             Law provides for applications, renewals, denials, suspensions and revocations,
                             reinstatement of certification, as well as for the collection of an annual fee for
                             certificate holders.

                             Law provides for annual inspection of each mammography system, and directs
                             facilities that fail this inspection to inform patients of the deficiencies and direct
                             them to another appropriate facility.

Effective Date   July 1, 1994; amended September 1, 1997.

Texas   TEX. INS. CODE ART. 21.52G

Scope   Reimbursement for Length of Stay/Inpatient Care Following Mastectomy

Policies   Law requires health insurers that provide coverage for breast cancer treatment to
and Limits   include coverage for inpatient care for an enrollee for a minimum of 48 hours
                     following a mastectomy, and 24 hours following a lymph node dissection. Law
                     states that health insurers are not required to provide the minimum hours of
                     coverage of inpatient care required if the attending physician of the enrollee
                     determines that a shorter period of inpatient care is appropriate.

                     Insurance plans may not deny an insured individual for the purpose of avoiding
                     the above requirements, provide monetary incentives for accepting less than these
                     requirements, penalize health care providers for providing care in accordance
                     with these requirements, or provide incentives to a provider to provide less than
                     the required care mandated by this law. In addition, insurers may not restrict
                     benefits for any portion of a hospital stay in a manner that is less favorable than
                     the benefits provided for any preceding portion of the stay.

                     Law requires insurers to provide notice, in writing, to enrollees regarding the
                     required coverage.

                     Law applies to individual, group, blanket, or franchise policies or agreements;
                     contracts issued by nonprofit hospital, or an individual or group evidence of
                     coverage that is offered by an insurance company, a group hospital service
                     corporation, a fraternal benefit society, a stipulated premium insurance company,
                     or a health maintenance organization. Law also applies to health benefit plans
                     that provide coverage only for a specific disease or condition or for
                     hospitalization.

                     Law does not apply to plans that provide coverage: (i) only for accidental death
                     or dismemberment; (ii) for wages or payments in lieu of wages for a period
                     during which an employee is absent from work because of sickness or injury; or
                     (iii) as a supplement to liability insurance. Law also does not apply to Medicare
                     supplemental policies, workers' compensation policies, medical payment
                     insurance issued as part of motor vehicle insurance policies, or long-term care
                     policies.

Quality Assurance Not indicated.

Effective Date   September 1, 1997

Utah   UTAH CODE ANN. §§ 26-21a-101 TO 26-21a-301

Scope   Accreditation of Facilities and Technologists/
                            Breast Cancer Screening and Education Programs

Policies   Law directs that the Utah Department of Health, in consultation with an advisory
and Limits   committee on mammogram quality assurance, make recommendations to the
                            Division of Occupational and Professional Licensing on rules establishing
                            qualifications and quality assurance standards for physician supervisors,
                            physicians interpreting mammograms, and radiological technologists.

                            A mammogram may only be performed at a facility certified by the Department.
                            The Department shall establish quality assurance standards for facilities
                            performing screening or diagnostic mammography or developing mammogram
                            X-ray films.

                            Law directs the Department to create a Breast Cancer Mortality Reduction
                            Program, which shall include:

                            # education programs for health professionals on skills in cancer screening,
                            diagnosis, referral, treatment, and rehabilitation based on current scientific
                            knowledge;

                            # education programs for the public on the benefits of regular breast cancer
                            screening; available resources for screening, diagnosis, referral, treatment and
                            rehabilitation; available treatment options; and

                            # subsidized screening programs for low-income women.

Effective Date   January 1, 1992. [Law applicable to § 26-21a-202 last amendment effective
                            April 29, 1996.]

Utah   UTAH CODE ANN. §§ 19-3-103.5, 19-3-104

Scope   Accreditation of Facilities

Policies   Law authorizes the state board responsible for radiation control to apply to the
and Limits   U.S. Food and Drug Administration for approval as an accrediting body under
                            the Mammography Quality Standards Act of 1992. Pursuant to such approval,
                            the board is authorized to accredit mammography facilities in accordance with
                            the Act, and to review and approve the qualifications of individuals who oversee
                            quality assurance at mammography facilities.

Effective Date   1995 enactment.

Vermont   8 V.S.A. § 4100a

Scope   Reimbursement for Breast Cancer Screening

Women's Age,   -50   Upon recommendation of the health care provider
Frequency of
Mammogram   50+   Each year

Policies   Law requires that insurers provide coverage for low-dose screening
and limits   mammograms for determining the presence of occult breast cancer.

                     Benefits must be at least as favorable as those provided for other radiological
                     examinations under the same policy, and shall be subject to the same dollar
                     limits, deductibles, and coinsurance factors.

                     Law does not apply to coverage for specified disease or other limited benefit
                     coverage.

                     Law defines "low-dose mammography" and "screening."

Quality Assurance After January 1, 1994, the law applies only to screening procedures conducted
                     by test facilities accredited by the American College of Radiologists.

Effective Date   January 2, 1991.

Vermont 18 V.S.A. § 157

Scope Mammography Registry

Policies
and limits Law requires a uniform statewide population-based registry system for the collection of mammography and pathology data relating to breast cancer and any associated identifying information acquired by the Vermont Mammography Registry.

Quality Assurance Not indicated.

Effective Date Last amendment effective April 15, 1994

NOTE: See 8 V.S.A. § 151 to 156 for applicable provisions.

Virginia VA. CODE ANN. § 38.2-3418.1

Scope Reimbursement for Breast Cancer Screening

Woman's Age,   35-39   Baseline
Frequency
of Mammogram   40-49   Every 2 years

50+   Each year

Physician referral required.

Policies Law requires that insurers provide coverage for low-dose screening
and Limits mammograms for determining the presence of occult breast cancer.

Law applies to individual or group accident and sickness insurance policies
providing hospital, medical and surgical, or major medical coverage on an
expense-incurred basis; corporations providing individual or group accident and
sickness subscription contracts; and health maintenance organizations.

Law does not apply to short-term travel, accident-only, limited or specified
disease policies, or short-term nonrenewable policies of up to 6 months duration.

Coverage may be limited to a benefit of $50 per mammogram, subject to dollar
limits, deductibles, and coinsurance factor no less favorable than for physical
illness generally.

Law defines "mammogram."

Quality Assurance Examination must use equipment dedicated specifically for mammography and
must meet Virginia Department of Health standards.

Examination must be performed by a registered technologist, interpreted by a
qualified radiologist, and performed under the direction of a person licensed to
practice medicine and surgery who is certified by the American College of
Radiology.

The facility must retain the mammography film in accordance with American
College of Radiology guidelines or Virginia law.

Effective Date 1990; last amendment effective July 1, 1996.

Virginia VA. CODE ANN. § 2.1-20.1(B)

Scope	Reimbursement for Breast Cancer Services for Public Employees	

Woman's Age, *Frequency* *of Mammogram*	35-39	Baseline
	40-49	Every two years
	50+	Each year

Policies
and Limits

Mammography:
Law requires that state employees' health insurance plan provide coverage for low-dose screening mammograms for determining the presence of occult breast cancer.

Coverage may be limited to a benefit of $50 per mammogram, subject to dollar limits, deductibles, and coinsurance factor no less favorable than for physical illness generally.

Treatment:
Law requires plan to cover the treatment of breast cancer by dose-intensive chemotherapy with autologous bone marrow transplants or stem cell support.

Reconstructive Surgery:
Law requires plan to include coverage for reconstructive breast surgery coincident with a mastectomy performed for breast cancer or following a mastectomy performed for breast cancer to reestablish symmetry between the two breasts (this provision is effective July 1, 1998).

Length of Stay Following Mastectomy:
Law requires plans to include coverage providing a minimum stay in the hospital of not less than 48 hours of inpatient care following a total mastectomy or partial mastectomy with lymph node dissection for treatment of breast cancer, expect when a shorter stay has been deemed sufficient by the physician in consultation with the patient.

Law defines "mammogram."

Quality Assurance   Examination must use equipment dedicated specifically for mammography. Mammograms must be ordered by a health care practitioner acting within the scope of his or her licensure, and in the care of an enrollee of a health maintenance organization, by the health maintenance organization physician; performed by a registered technologist; interpreted by a qualified radiologist; and performed under the direction of a person licensed to practice medicine or surgery and certified by the American Board of Radiology or an equivalent examining body. In addition, a copy of the mammogram must be sent to the health care practitioner who ordered it, and the equipment used must meet standards set forth by the Virginia Department of Health in its radiation protection standards.

Covered treatments must be performed by clinical programs authorized to provide such therapies under clinical trials sponsored by the National Cancer Institute.

Effective Date   1984 enactment; amended March 18, 1995.

Virginia   VA. CODE ANN. § 32.1-325

Scope   Reimbursement for Breast Cancer Treatment for Recipients of Medical
                        Assistance

Policies   Law requires a payment of medical assistance to cover the treatment of breast
and Limits   cancer (or lymphoma) in individuals over the age of 21 by high-dose
                        chemotherapy and bone marrow transplants if they have been determined by the
                        treating health care provider to have a performance status sufficient to proceed
                        with such treatment.

                        Law provides that appeals of these cases shall be handled in accordance with the
                        health department's expedited appeals process.

Quality Assurance   Not indicated.

Effective Date   280 Days from March 21, 1997.

Virginia VA. CODE ANN. § 54.1-2971

Scope Alternative Therapies/Informed Consent for Treatment of Breast Cancer

Policies Law requires the execution of a consent form before a physician operates on a
and Limits patient for a breast tumor.

The consent form must include the following:

"CONSENT FOR TREATMENT OF BREAST TUMOR"

Sign option (a) or option (b), or option (a) and option (b).

(a) I authorize Dr.................... to perform a Breast Biopsy
....
Side (right and/or left)

....
Patient's or other authorized person's signature

(b) If it is determined that I have a malignant tumor in my breast or other
breast abnormality requiring surgery, then I authorize Dr.................... to
perform such operations or procedures, including breast removal, which are
deemed necessary.

Procedure:
....
....
Patient's or other authorized person's signature

Quality Assurance Not indicated.

Effective Date 1984 enactment.

Virginia   VA. CODE ANN. § 38.2-3418.1:1

Scope   Reimbursement for Chemotherapy and Bone Marrow Transplant for Breast
                 Cancer

Policies   Law requires insurers to provide coverage for the treatment of cancer by dose-
and Limits   intensive chemotherapy/autologous bone marrow transplants or stem cell
                    transplants.

                    The coverage shall not be subject to any greater copayment than that applicable
                    to any other coverage provided by such policies, and the coverage shall be
                    subject to the same deductible as that applicable to other coverage. A deductible
                    for this coverage in a different amount may, however, be offered and made
                    available.

                    Law applies to accident and sickness policies providing hospital, medical and
                    surgical, or major medical coverage on an expense-incurred basis; accident and
                    sickness subscription contracts; and health maintenance organizations.

                    Law does not apply to short-term travel, accident-only, limited or specified
                    disease policies or short-term, nonrenewable policies of less than 6 months'
                    duration.

Quality Assurance   Treatment must be performed pursuant to protocols approved by the institutional
                        review board of any United States medical teaching college including, but not
                        limited to National Cancer Institute protocols that have been favorably reviewed
                        and utilized by hematologists or oncologists experiences in these treatments.

Effective Date   January 1, 1995.

Virginia   VA. CODE ANN. § 38.2-3418.4

Scope   Reimbursement for Breast Reconstruction or Prosthesis

Policies   Law requires that each insurer issuing an individual or group accident or
and Limits   insurance policy providing a health care plan or health care services shall provide
                                coverage for reconstructive breast surgery.

                                Law does not apply to short-term travel, accident only, limited or specified
                                disease policies (except policies issued for cancer), Medicare policies or
                                contracts, or any other similar coverage under state and federal governmental
                                plans or to short-term nonrenewable policies of not more than 6 months'
                                duration.

                                The reimbursement for reconstructive breast surgery shall be determined
                                according to the same formula by which charges are developed for other medical
                                and surgical procedures. Such coverage shall have durational limits, dollar limits,
                                deductibles, and coinsurance factors that are no less favorable than for physical
                                illness generally.

                                Law defines "mastectomy" and "reconstructive breast surgery."

Quality Assurance   Not indicated.

Effective Date   July 1, 1998.

VA. CODE ANN. § 38.2-3418.6

Scope

Reimbursement for Length of Stay Following Mastectomy

Policies and Limits

Law requires that each insurer issuing an individual or group accident or insurance policy shall provide coverage for a minimum stay in the hospital of not less than 48 hours for a patient following a radical or modified mastectomy, and not less than 24 hours of inpatient care following a total mastectomy or a partial mastectomy with lymph node dissection for the treatment of breast cancer, except when a shorter stay has been deemed sufficient by the physician in consultation with the patient.

This law does not apply to short-term travel; accident only; limited or specified disease policies; policies or contracts designed for issuance to persons eligible for coverage under Medicare; or any other similar coverage under state or federal government plans, or to short-term non-renewable policies of not more than 6 months' duration.

Quality Assurance

Not indicated.

Effective Date

July 1, 1998.

| Virginia | **2000 Va. ALS 319; 2000 Va. Acts 319;** |
| | **2000 Va. Ch. 319; 2000 Va. HB 722** |

Scope   Special License Plates Supporting Breast Cancer Screening and Research

Policies   Law authorizes the issuance of special license plates bearing the legend "Virginia
and Limits   Breast Cancer Foundation."

Law states that the special plates shall be issued upon the payment of the
prescribed fee for state license plates and an additional annual fee of $25. For
each such $25 fee collected in excess of 1,000 registrations, $15 shall be
deposited to the credit of the Virginia Breast Cancer Foundation Fund and shall
be used to support statewide breast cancer educational programs.

Quality Assurance   Not indicated.

Effective Date   April 3, 2000

Washington   **RCW §§ 41.05.180, 48.20.393, 48.21.225,**
                        48.44.325, 48.46.275

Scope   Reimbursement for Breast Cancer Screening

Woman's Age,   Not stipulated.
Frequency
of Mammogram   Recommendation by physician, advanced nurse practitioner, or physician's
                        assistant required.

Policies   Law requires that insurance policies providing coverage for hospital or medical
and Limits   expenses provide coverage for screening or diagnostic mammography.

                        Law applies to disability insurance policies, group disability policies, health care
                        service contracts, health maintenance organizations, and public employee health
                        plans.

                        Law does not apply to Medicare supplement policies or supplemental contracts
                        covering specified disease or other limited benefits.

                        Law does not prevent the application of standard policy provisions such as
                        copayment or deductible provisions applicable to other benefits. Law does not
                        limit insurer's authority to negotiate with providers for delivery of mammography
                        services.

Quality Assurance   Not indicated.

Effective Date   January 1, 1990; last amended 1994.

Washington	**RCW §§ 48.20.395, 48.21.230,** **48.44.330, 48.46.280**

Scope Reimbursement for Breast Reconstruction and Prosthesis

Policies Law requires that insurers provide benefits for reconstructive breast surgery
and Limits resulting from a mastectomy that resulted from disease, illness, or injury.

Law applies to disability insurance policies, group disability policies, health care service contracts, and health maintenance organizations.

Law (as amended effective January 1, 1986) also requires that insurers provide coverage for all stages of one reconstructive breast reduction on the non-diseased breast to make it equal in size with the diseased breast after definitive reconstructive surgery.

Quality Assurance Not indicated.

Effective Date July 24, 1983; last amendment effective January 1, 1986.

Washington   **RCW §§ 48.20.397, 48.21.235, 48.44.335, 48.46.285**

Scope   Restrictions on Denial of Insurance Coverage for Breast Cancer Survivors

Policies   Law states that no insurer may refuse to issue, cancel, or decline to renew a
and Limits   contract or policy solely because of a mastectomy or lumpectomy performed on
       the insured more than 5 years previously.

       Law prohibits any restriction, modification, exclusion, increase, or reduction in
       the amount of benefits payable, or any term, rate, condition, or type of coverage
       solely based on a mastectomy or lumpectomy performed on the insured more
       than 5 years previously.

Quality Assurance   Not indicated.

Effective Date   January 1, 1986.

West Virginia   W.VA. CODE §§ 16-33-1 to 16-33-12

Scope   Breast Cancer Screening and Education Programs/
Fund for Breast Cancer Diagnosis and Treatment

Policies   *Breast and Cervical Cancer Detection and Education Program:*
and Limits   Law establishes the Breast and Cervical Cancer Detection and Education
Program. The program is established to promote screening and detection of
breast and cervical cancers among unserved or underserved populations, to
educate the public regarding breast and cervical cancers and the benefits of early
detection, and to provide counseling and referral services.

The West Virginia Director of Health shall make grants to approved
organizations for the provision of services relating to the screening and detection
of breast and cervical cancers.

Law creates the Breast and Cervical Cancer Detection and Education Program
Coalition to advise the Director. The Director shall report annually to the
Governor and Legislature concerning the operation of the program.

Breast and Cervical Cancer Diagnostic and Treatment Fund:
Law establishes the Breast and Cervical Cancer Diagnostic and Treatment Fund
for the care of indigent patients requiring diagnostic or treatment services for
breast or cervical cancer.

The Fund shall be administered by the Office of Maternal and Child Health
within the Bureau of Public Health, and may include moneys appropriated by the
Legislature or received from the federal government or other public and private
sources.

Procedures and requirements for use of the Fund shall be established by the
medical advisory committee of the Breast and Cervical Cancer Detection and
Education Program Coalition.

To be financially eligible for services reimbursed by the Fund, a patient cannot
be covered by Medicaid, Medicare, or other medical insurance, and must have an
income at or below 200 percent of the federal poverty level. To be medically
eligible for diagnostic services, a patient must have a condition strongly
suspicious of cancer and need diagnostic services to confirm a preliminary
diagnosis. A positive pathology report is required to be eligible for treatment
services.

The Fund is the payor of last resort. Payments for services shall be at the
prevailing rates established by Medicare.

Quality Assurance   Not indicated.

Effective Date   July 1, 1992; amended in 1996.

West Virginia   **W.Va. Code §§ 33-15-4c, 33-16-3g, 33-24-7b, 33-25-8a, 33-25A-8a**

Scope   Reimbursement for Breast Cancer Screening

Woman's Age,   35-39   Baseline
Frequency
of Mammogram   40-49   Every 2 years, or more frequently upon physician's
                                    recommendation

                       50+   Each year

                       Physician's referral required.

Policies   Law requires that insurance policies covering laboratory or X-ray services also
and Limits   cover mammograms.

                       Law applies to individual and group accident and sickness policies; health
                       maintenance organizations; health care corporations; and hospital, medical,
                       dental, and health service corporations.

                       The insurer may apply the same deductibles, coinsurance, and other limitations
                       as apply to other covered services.

Quality Assurance   Not indicated.

Effective Date   July 1, 1989.

West Virginia   **W.VA. CODE §§ 5-16-7, 5-16-9**

Scope   Reimbursement for Breast Cancer Screening for Public Employees

Woman's Age,   35-39   Baseline
Frequency
of Mammogram   40-49   Every 2 years, or as needed

                       50+   Every year

Policies   Law requires that the health insurance plan for public employees provide
and Limits   coverage for X-ray services in connection with mammograms performed for
                       cancer screening or diagnostic purposes.

                       The plan covers employees of state agencies and county boards of education, as
                       well as employees of participating counties, cities, towns, and other public
                       agencies.

Quality Assurance   Not indicated.

Effective Date   Last amended April 1, 1996.

Wisconsin   **WIS. STAT. § 255.06**

Scope   Breast Cancer Screening and Education Programs

Policies   Law establishes the Breast Cancer Screening Program. The program provides
and Limits   grants for women 40 years and older residing in the 12 rural counties with the
                       highest incidence of late-stage breast cancer.

                       The state makes grants to approved hospitals or organizations that have available
                       mammography units for use in the service areas. The amount of payment for
                       services depends upon the income-level and availability of third-party payment.

Quality Assurance   Not indicated.

Effective Date   1991; last amended 1997.

Wisconsin   WIS. STAT. § 632.895(8)

Scope   Reimbursement for Breast Cancer Screening

Woman's Age,   45-49   Two examinations
Frequency
of Mammogram   50+   Each year

                      Physician's or nurse practitioner's referral required, with specified exceptions.

Policies   Law requires that disability insurance policies provide coverage for low-dose
and Limits   mammography to screen for the presence of breast cancer.

                      Law applies to surgical, medical, hospital, major medical, or other health service
                      coverage.

                      Law does not apply to policies covering specified diseases, limited service health
                      organization plans, Medicare replacement policies, Medicare supplement
                      policies, and long-term care policies.

                      Coverage may only be subject to exclusions and limitations that apply to other
                      radiological examinations.

                      Law defines "low-dose mammography."

Quality Assurance   Examination must use equipment dedicated specifically for mammography.

Effective Date   March 31, 1990.

| **Wisconsin** | WIS. STAT. § 632.895(8) |

Scope Reimbursement for Breast Reconstruction or Prosthesis

Policies and Limits Law requires every disability insurance policy and every self-insured health plan of the state of Wisconsin that provides coverage of the surgical procedure known as a mastectomy to also provide coverage of breast reconstruction of the affected tissue incident to a mastectomy.

Coverage may be subject to any exclusions, limitations or cost-sharing provisions that apply generally under the disability insurance policy or self-insured health plan.

Quality Assurance Not indicated.

Effective Date March 31, 1990.

Wyoming   WYO. STAT. §§ 26-18-103, 26-19-107

Scope   Reimbursement for Breast Cancer Screening

Woman's Age,   Not stipulated
Frequency
of Mammogram

Policies   Law requires individual and group insurance policies issued or delivered on or
and Limits   after January 1, 1999 to disclose (on the face of the policy in type of no less than
                   14 point bold) the extent to which the policy includes comprehensive adult
                   wellness benefits, including testing for breast cancer.

                   Benefits are not subject to policy deductibles and must provide a minimum
                   benefit equal to 80 percent of the reimbursement allowance under the private
                   health benefit plan with a maximum of 20 percent coinsurance by the insured and
                   which provide a benefit structure to the insured equal to a minimum of $150 per
                   insured adult per calender year.

Quality Assurance Not stipulated.

Effective Date   Last amendment effective July 1, 1998.

INDEX

www.ingramcontent.com/pod-product-compliance
Lightning Source LLC
Chambersburg PA
CBHW080240180526
45167CB00006B/2351